I0606206

PRAISE FOR *UNBLINDED*

"As an empathetic, highly responsible ophthalmology resident at the Wilmer Eye Institute at Johns Hopkins in the late 1980s, Dr. David Guyer was unhappy that so many of his older patients were suffering from the visually disabling disease known as Age-related Macular Degeneration (AMD). Like so many of his colleagues, and even his teachers and their own forebears, Dr. Guyer was taught to politely and gently tell his patients, 'I am so sorry, but there is nothing I can do.'

It was a problem previously thought to be unsolvable. However, Dr. Guyer with only a few collaborating young ophthalmologists, within only a few years after finishing their training, cofounded a new biotech company (Eyetech, Inc.). There, they discovered a new class of chemical compounds known as 'anti-VEGFs,' including Macugen, which amazingly improved AMD, and obtained FDA approval to market this novel therapeutic agent in the United States. It represented a significant, life-altering achievement.

Unblinded tells the story of this monumental achievement and provides readers the inspirational, heartwarming story of insight, imagination, perseverance, and intellectual brilliance that characterized Dr. Guyer and his team.

Not only was their innovative therapy successful in reversing and preventing blindness from AMD, it also stimulated an avalanche of important, and ultimately successful, pharmacological research for a wide variety of other blinding eye diseases, including diabetic retinopathy, thrombosed retinal veins, retinal detachments, as well as for AMD and others.

If the famous scientist, Louis Pasteur, had been alive to consider the story of Dr. Guyer and his dedicated colleagues, he would have been impressed, reassured, and very proud of each of them."

—MORTON F. GOLDBERG, MD, DIRECTOR EMERITUS, WILMER EYE INSTITUTE AND PROFESSOR OF OPHTHALMOLOGY, JOHNS HOPKINS SCHOOL OF MEDICINE

"Generations will continue to benefit from David Guyer's vision and passion to combat one of the leading causes of blindness, age-related macular degeneration. Guyer helped to spark a global quest among retinal specialists, biopharmaceutical companies, and Wall Street that will continue to save countless people from losing their vision."

—MICHAEL GAITO, GLOBAL CHAIRMAN OF INVESTMENT BANKING AND HEALTHCARE, J.P. MORGAN

"*Unblinded* shares the vital story of the struggle and ultimate success in developing anti-VEGF—one of the most important breakthroughs ever in ophthalmology—a crucial drug for patients that saved sight for millions.

In 2000, David Guyer, Tony Adamis, and Samir Patel founded Eyetech. As CEO, David showed great talent and initiative, acquiring a unique anti-VEGF agent, Macugen (pegaptanib sodium), raising the needed funding, and building the teams for clinical trials, manufacturing, and regulatory approval. The approval of Macugen changed the way we treat patients with retinal disease and paved the way for multiple anti-VEGF therapies, which are now given to millions of patients around the world every year. The blindness burden worldwide has been lessened because of these treatments.

It is hard to describe the thrill of that moment—taking findings in the laboratory to patients and developing a successful clinical treatment. None of us expected our early work to lead to such a revolution in patient care."

—JOAN MILLER, MD, MASSACHUSETTS EYE AND EAR, CHAIR OF OPHTHALMOLOGY; HARVARD MEDICAL SCHOOL CHAIR OF THE DEPARTMENT OF OPHTHALMOLOGY, DAVID GLENDENNING COGAN PROFESSOR OF OPHTHALMOLOGY

"Losing your vision is as emotional a condition as having cancer. Mechanistically, because of neovascularization, one can call wet AMD a cancer of the eye. It is in that context that we all need to think of the contributions to medicine that David Guyer, Tony Adamis, and Samir Patel have made with their pioneering work at Eyetech."

—NICHOLAS GALAKATOS, GLOBAL HEAD OF LIFE SCIENCES, BLACKSTONE

"Whether it arrives from an act of nature, serendipity, or inspired creation, an important beginning is fascinating to study. Some beginnings can be chronicled with crystal clarity while others are imprecise or even contentious, giving rise to discussions that breathe additional life into our interest. However, if the beginning gives rise to a trend that is a profoundly significant one, it is paradoxically at high risk of being unappreciated and forgotten.

The story of Vascular Endothelial Growth Factor (VEGF) also has a beginning, and it is both intricate and fascinating. Intravitreal injection of anti-VEGF agents has become the most common non-diagnostic ophthalmic procedure and has completely transformed retinal practice with its runaway success in treating a variety of iconic retinal diseases.

Unblinded explores the fascinating origins of our anti-VEGF agents as the first retinal pharmaceuticals and gives an insider's account of the physicians and scientists who progressively encircled VEGF—stepwise and relentlessly, like a group of hunters pursuing a wolf through dark woods—as a principal agent of so much visual loss and human suffering. If we look even closer, the VEGF story is nothing less than the birth of true retinal pharmacology, a pivotal moment in our specialty that like all beginnings, is populated with discoveries, luck, events, and most importantly, people.

David, as my retina fellow during 1990–92, transformed from a consummate academic retina specialist (he could write an original and luminous medical manuscript in a day!) to the single most savvy retinal pharmaceutical CEO in history. His instincts regarding which targets were worth pursuing (that is, buying the rights to and developing companies around, often as a gamble) and which to pass over are a result of a process impenetrable to observers, and I keep it in the same mental folder as the successful divination of well water with a forked stick. Combined with his high-octane energy and management skills, a winning target was certain to become an FDA-approved drug. He would go on to become an insightful retinal venture capitalist and serial entrepreneur, sharing his successes with numerous colleagues and coworkers. Remarkably, he shows no signs of stopping or even slowing down, and savvy retina specialists would do well to keep his heels within view."

—DONALD J. D'AMICO, MD, JOHN MILTON MCLEAN PROFESSOR AND CHAIR, WEILL CORNELL MEDICINE OPHTHALMOLOGY; OPHTHALMOLOGIST-IN-CHIEF, NEWYORK-PRESBYTERIAN HOSPITAL

"David Guyer founded Eyetech and pioneered the development of Macugen. This therapeutic approach is among the most important innovations in ophthalmology during the past 50 years. Anti-VEGF therapy has enabled millions of patients to remain gainfully employed and lead independent lives. David Guyer's work has had a major impact on reducing blindness among millions of patients."

—MARCO A. ZARBIN, MD, PHD, PROFESSOR AND CHAIR, INSTITUTE OF OPHTHALMOLOGY AND VISUAL SCIENCE, RUTGERS NEW JERSEY MEDICAL SCHOOL

amplify
an imprint of Amplify Publishing Group

UNBLINDED

The Start-Up That Launched a Revolution in Saving Sight

DAVID R. GUYER, MD
and IAN KELDOULIS

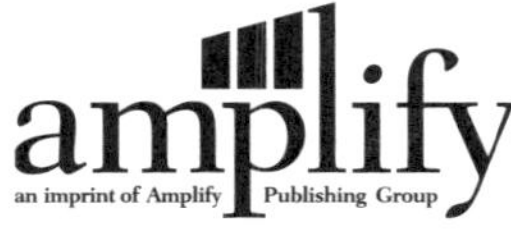

www.amplifypublishinggroup.com

Unblinded: The Start-Up That Launched a Revolution in Saving Sight

For more information, please contact:
Amplify Publishing, an imprint of Amplify Publishing Group
620 Herndon Parkway, Suite 220
Herndon, VA 20170
info@amplifypublishing.com

Library of Congress Control Number: 2025919181

CPSIA Code: PRV0925A

ISBN-13: 979-8-89138-871-0

Printed in the United States

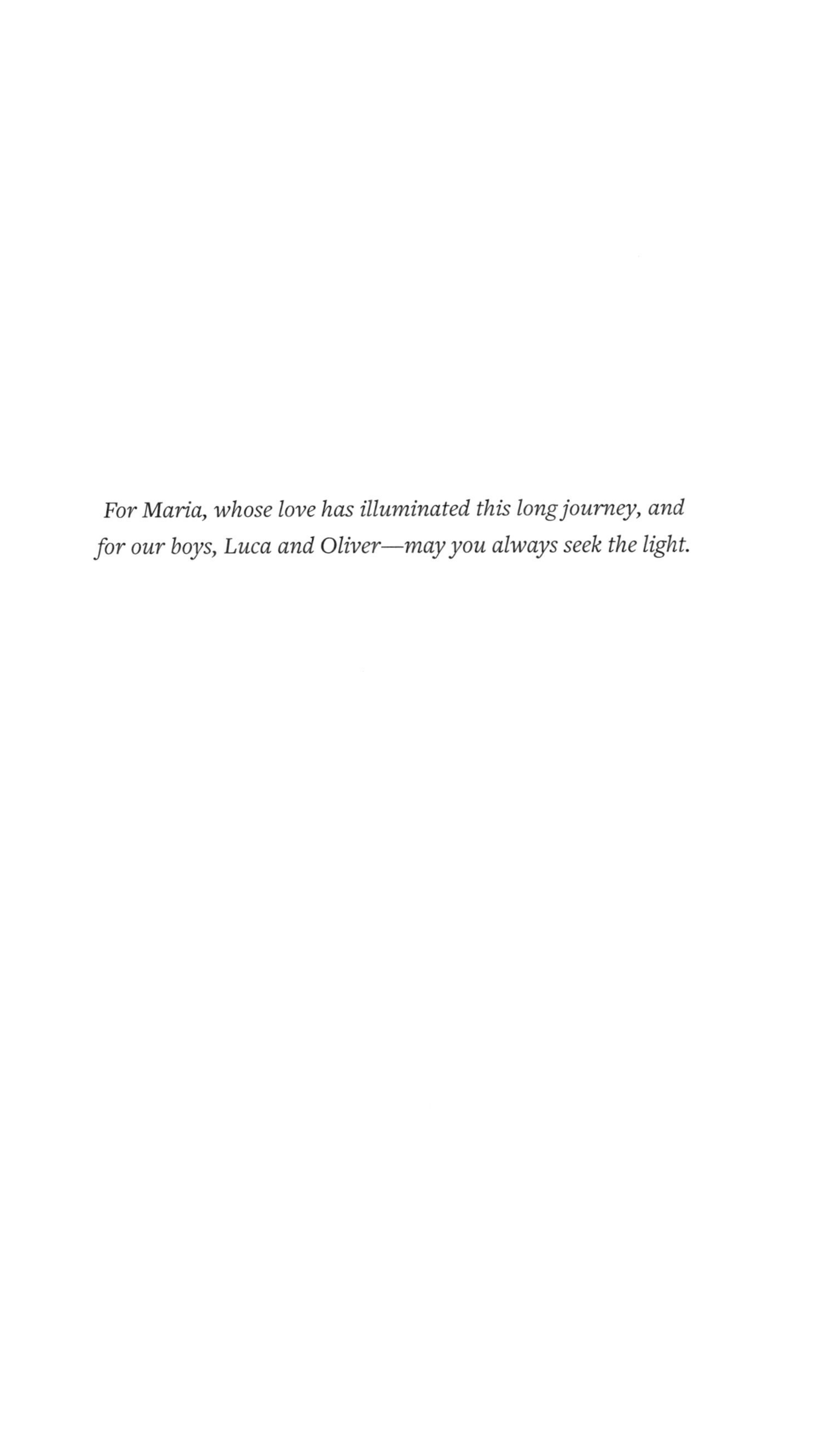

For Maria, whose love has illuminated this long journey, and for our boys, Luca and Oliver—may you always seek the light.

CONTENTS

FOREWORD

There are very few moments in biotech—perhaps in medicine as a whole—when everything changes. When a disease that once meant irreversible decline suddenly becomes manageable. Treatable. Even reversible. For millions of people living with wet age-related macular degeneration, that moment arrived with the approval of Macugen®. And it happened because of David Guyer, MD.

I first met David in the early days of Eyetech Pharmaceuticals, when SV first backed David in early 2000. At the time, there were no drugs for wet AMD. The prognosis for patients—many of them elderly, many just beginning to lose their central vision—was devastating. You could offer laser treatment, maybe, or prepare patients for low-vision aids. But the basic truth was they were going to go blind.

What David and his team, including Tony Adamis and Samir Patel, did at Eyetech changed that forever. What followed was a masterclass in biotech value creation. With Macugen, they delivered not just a drug, but a turning point. For the first time, physicians had a way to intervene pharmacologically—early, precisely, and with the possibility of preserving or even restoring vision. Macugen® was the first-ever anti-VEGF treatment for wet AMD. It's hard to overstate the impact of that moment. For patients, it meant regaining the ability to read, to drive, to recognize a loved one's face. For families, it meant holding on to independence, dignity, connection.

It was the first time in history you could treat vision loss with a drug. Not a laser. A drug. It worked. People started seeing again.

Behind that breakthrough was David's vision. As a retina specialist, he didn't just understand the biology; he lived the clinical reality. He had spent years delivering hard news to patients and was determined to change the story. David also surrounded himself with brilliant people who passionately shared David's vision. That's what gave Eyetech its urgency, its clarity of purpose, and its credibility. Investors followed not just the science, but the mission. We believed in what David was building because we saw firsthand the scale of human suffering he was trying to address.

And he delivered. Eyetech went public, Macugen was approved, and the field of ophthalmology was transformed. Anti-VEGF therapy became the foundation of care for wet AMD, and everything that came after—Lucentis, Eylea, Vabysmo—built on the ground that David helped to break open. A $22 billion-a-year therapeutic class was born. Guyer didn't just bring a drug to market—he created a market. That's the kind of move investors call platform potential, and biotech strategists call once-in-a-generation.

But he wasn't done.

Guyer kept building and brought his gang, including Samir, Evelyn Harrison, and Loni da Silva, back together for a second venture in 2007: Ophthotech, later Iveric Bio, which again SV backed. Following the clinical setback of the Fovista trials in 2016, David convinced the board to prioritize the second program in geographic atrophy, Zimura (avacincaptad pegol), later known as Izervay. This yielded tangible results, delivering successful pivotal Phase 3 data showing an approximately 30 percent slowing of GA progression. This trial set the stage for Iveric Bio's multi-billion-dollar acquisition by Astellas. A transaction that again powerfully validated Guyer's strategic vision and his ability to turn setbacks into substantial patient and shareholder gains.

In 2021 David's entrepreneurial itch returned, and he worked with our team at SV to create EyeBio. David quietly assembled another crackerjack team, including Tony as a cofounder, Sarah Milsom as chief operating officer, Jon Prenner as chief medical officer (CMO), Samir for critical input, and once again his longtime collaborator Evelyn onto the board. They skipped the noise, focused on first-in-class science, and built real momentum with their WNT agonist lead asset before anyone outside the loop realized what was happening. Less than three years later, Merck stepped in with a $3 billion offer. It looked effortless, but it was classic Guyer: clinical clarity, strategic timing, and a nose for what actually matters.

But for me, Eyetech is the origin story. It's where we saw just how much could be achieved when a brilliant clinician with a clear sense of purpose takes on an unmet need with the tools of modern biotechnology.

So what do we, as investors, take away from this?

First: de-risked innovation is real—and rare. Guyer didn't chase shiny objects; he found neglected biology with clear endpoints and deep clinical need. Second: clinical credibility scales. Physician-scientists like him don't just think differently; they design better trials, pick smarter indications, recruit expert, loyal teams, and carry trust into every boardroom and partnering meeting. Third: the societal dividend matters. Because the reason this all worked wasn't just the science—it was the problem. Retinal blindness in an aging world isn't a niche. It's a ticking public health bomb. And David Guyer defused it.

While the rest of us were busy backing CRISPR companies with preclinical mouse data, he quietly built three of the most successful ophthalmic companies of our time. This book tells you how. From the inside. It's a founder's tale, but also an investor's road map. A case study in how to spot asymmetric bets that happen to save lives.

The best biotech investments are those where everyone wins. Where shareholders see returns, certainly—but where patients experience something even more profound: the return of hope. That's what David Guyer gave the world with Eyetech. He didn't just build a company. He gave people their sight back.

And what could matter more than that?

—Dame Kate Bingham, managing partner, SV Health Investors, and chair of the UK Vaccine Taskforce during the Covid-19 pandemic reporting directly to the Prime Minister.

INTRODUCTION

This book is about a revolution. A revolution heralding one of the most life-enhancing discoveries of all time that has ended suffering for millions of people. Yet, ironically, for the general public, this revolution has been largely invisible for 20 years. How is that possible in the information age, you might wonder?

For a generation, we've been accustomed to disruption on a daily basis, a trend that's accelerating. So, why did this incredible breakthrough get overlooked? In our youth-focused culture, when a revolution impacts the elderly—in this case literally illuminating their golden years—society isn't equipped to publicize it. And when we avert a crisis before it happens, the headlines never get written, there are no videos to go viral. Good news is no news. In short, the fact that our world isn't overrun with blind old people is something we take for granted. But at the turn of this century, that was not the case at all. We were on the cusp of a social catastrophe.

In 2000, when Eyetech, the company at the center of this book, was founded, there were 40 million Americans aged 65 and older. By 2020, this number had grown to almost 56 million, 16.8% of the population. In most other advanced nations this percentage is even higher. In the ten years between 2010 and 2020, the growth rate of the elderly in the US outpaced the general population by a factor of five. A study published in the *Journal of the American Medical Association* (JAMA) Ophthalmology in 2022 estimated that around 20 million Americans had age-related macular degeneration (AMD). As it progresses, AMD robs you of your central vision. The report makes clear that the older you get, particularly past 75, the more your chance of severe visual impairment escalates dramatically. The most routine things become extremely challenging or impossible. Reading, writing, recognizing faces, preparing food, driving, the list goes on. Without the treatments pioneered by the doctors and researchers in this book, our newfound longevity would be marred by our inability to function. Instead of old people enjoying retirement, they would be almost completely dependent on others.

Of course, this revolution affects the young and the middle-aged, too. Millennials and especially Gen X, without realizing it, have gained hours daily to pursue their goals. This gift is the time they would otherwise be spending taking care of their blind, elderly relatives. And even the youngest generation benefits from having great-grandparents who can recognize them and read them bedtime stories.

Three eye doctors are at the center of this revolution: Dr. David Guyer, a New York academic and prolific writer of papers; Dr. Tony Adamis, a researcher in Boston inspired by studies of tumor growth; and Dr. Samir Patel, a leading Chicago-based surgeon. This is the story of how they forever altered eye care. Together, they refocused the attention of the pharmaceutical industry from the front of the eye to the back. What may seem like a simple anatomical shift of a few millimeters has had a profound impact. Not only has the industry moved beyond devising drops to reduce irritation and redness, but it has also opened up a $15 billion+ annual market for retinal disease treatments injected directly into the eyeball. Now, these treatments are among the leading procedures reimbursed under Medicare Part B in the US.

How did this transformation come about? This book uncovers the seeds of discontent—the dissatisfaction with existing treatments, especially the false promise of the bright and shiny laser technology in the 1980s and '90s when everything *Star Wars* was in vogue. It witnesses the sparks of inspiration when breakthroughs in one area of medicine are repurposed for ophthalmology. Like all change, there are numerous obstacles and institutional resistance to overcome while support must be marshalled. And of course, revolutions need to be financed, too. With drug development, the stakes are spectacularly high.

This is also the story of personal metamorphosis. Not only did David, Tony, and Samir escape the confines of their profession, but they also had to learn on the fly how business operates, making their dreams real through concrete actions. Their success has led to the opening of entirely new career paths for eye doctors. The wall between academic ophthalmology and pharmaceuticals has been razed, allowing new medical approaches to be more readily developed.

Naturally, David, Tony, and Samir didn't do it alone. This book is the culmination of over fifty-five hours of conversations with dozens of fellow doctors, researchers, financiers, and company employees.

We hope it gives you a deeper understanding of what it takes to create enduring change: dedication, perseverance, a huge amount of luck, and most importantly, the knowledge of what to do when good fortune strikes.

Chapter 1

THREE STRIKES

Even with the jet stream behind him, it was a long flight back to New York. Despite rising above the clouds, Dr. David Guyer was at an all-time low. As a professor and the future chairman of the Department of Ophthalmology at New York University, David had built an impressive career. He graduated summa cum laude and Phi Beta Kappa in biology from Yale, attended medical school and completed his residency at Johns Hopkins, and finished a fellowship at Harvard Medical School. Failure was not something he was accustomed to.

Gnawing at the driven, self-assured eye doctor as he watched the vastness of the country steadily pass below wasn't his personal failure to reach an agreement with Genentech, the Bay Area biotech giant. Business wasn't his forte, after all. (Not yet at least.) What bothered him was the profound feeling that modern medicine, even its latest high-tech manifestation, was failing his patients. And every other eye specialist's patients, too. Millions of people were going blind. If he was right, their awful fate could be avoided.

* * *

What David was accustomed to—something which troubled him deeply—was routinely telling many of his older patients, "I'm very sorry; there's nothing I can do for you." It was a mantra familiar to all retina specialists, one that signaled the onset of a disease that would upend a person's life. Age-related macular degeneration (AMD) was the leading cause of blindness in the US and throughout the world wherever people's life expectancy was steadily increasing. For many elderly folks their golden years were tarnished by the loss of sight, a dark curtain descending on their hopes, draining their vitality, and rendering them utterly dependent on others. In 1996, when David met with Genentech, around the world more than half a million people over the age of fifty-five were getting the disease every year.

AMD is a stealthy disease, often unnoticeable at first. Eventually, a person detects subtle changes in their vision, and things start to get a little blurry—enough to make someone seek a new glasses prescription from their eye doctor. But unlike the usual culprits behind spectacles—nearsightedness, farsightedness, and astigmatism, caused by difficulty focusing light from the front of the eye to the rear—AMD affects the macula, the very center of your vision, located at the center of the retina, the screen of tissue at the back of the eye where light is transformed into the electrical impulses our brains need to create images. Think of it this way: The eye is the camera, and the retina is the film of the eye.

The debilitating disease comes in two forms: *dry*, or atrophic AMD, when the macula thins with age, and *wet*, otherwise known as neovascular AMD. Wet AMD is faster moving and more damaging, and it can develop from the dry form. With wet AMD, unlike in the slew of visual problems that manifest in the front of the eye, vision is undone by tiny malfunctioning blood vessels that leak, bleed, and eventually scar, destroying the macula, the area responsible for your central vision. Like old, eroded pipes leaking in your ceiling, the damage spreads outward from the middle. This means everything in front of you dims, while peripheral vision holds steady. If unchecked, the disease makes it increasingly challenging to focus and make out images. The ability to do essential activities like reading, recognizing faces, and driving becomes impaired. Eventually, in the worst cases, vision becomes nothing but a dark void, rimmed with light. For doctors used to the joy that improved sight gives to patients of all ages and the gratification of helping people enrich their lives—i.e., reading more easily; clearly seeing their loved ones smile; enjoying movies, art, and sunsets; and navigating the world effortlessly—diagnosing a patient with AMD was always delivered with dread. A sad conclusion to a life well lived.

Desperation was a hallmark of AMD sufferers. The elderly victims of the disease would, as the Welsh poet Dylan Thomas invoked in his most famous verse, "rage, rage, against the dying of the light." This took on many extreme manifestations. From buying all manner of arcane optical devices for enlarging objects in the line of sight to ingesting a litany of snake-oil remedies, patients would try anything that offered a faint glimmer of hope.

One case that particularly stuck in David's mind was that of a seventy-five-year-old gentleman named Tom. Tom had stumbled on the notion that spinach contained exactly the right kind of nutrients to reverse his progressive condition. Chock full of fiber, the leafy green is also packed with vitamins A and C, as well as iron, folate, and potassium. And one hundred grams of it will give you almost 2.9 grams of protein. It's really hard to say something bad about the vegetable. And there's little doubt that vitamin A in particular is associated with eye wellness. But despite all its health benefits, spinach does nothing to address the wayward vascular processes at the back of the eye that cause macular degeneration.

But those in deep despair find little solace in logic. For Tom, spinach promised transformation. The more he ate of it, the better. And he did eat it. Constantly. Five to seven bags of raw spinach daily was his preferred dose. He would show up to David's practice munching the stuff, affably chewing away in the waiting room. While there was a good chance this ravenous habit kept Tom's bowel movements regular, David saw no evidence that it did a lick of good for the back of his eyes. Ultimately, Tom's behavior came across as cartoonish, evoking a pitiable Popeye the Sailor Man—minus the magical effects of spinach.

* * *

While the reasons why Genentech wasn't open to considering David's request weren't readily apparent, the resistance was. At Genentech, David was confronted by what seemed to be a completely different lack of vision. One that aroused a full set of emotions, none of them positive. He'd crossed the country with the hope of taking a new molecule that Genentech was developing for oncology and deploying it for ophthalmic use. He felt this new genetically engineered molecule displayed tremendous potential to stop the blood vessels at the back of the eye from bleeding, arresting wet AMD. However, Genentech resolutely didn't see things the same way. Especially not the company's executives who met with him. It seemed as if they were mostly commercial people, focused on maximizing the drug's market potential, which meant using it for cancer. Everybody knew that's where the real money was.

But that wasn't the biggest obstacle to getting them on board. Ophthalmology was certainly way off their radar, but there was one thing about eyes they claimed to know all too well and unequivocally stated: Nobody, in their right mind, was going to get an injection directly into their eyeball. Over and over again. Every month. For the rest of their lives. David's treatment plan sounded like something straight out of a B-horror movie. The public would never buy it in a million years, no matter what it cost.

David fought hard. He knew his science. His knowledge was backed up by years of writing peer-reviewed papers on ophthalmology, possibly more during his medical training than almost anyone in the history of ophthalmology. And he was a master of persuasion. His communication skills were nothing less than stellar, honed in clinical practice, explaining complex medical situations to his patients in ways they could readily understand, and as a professor, enlightening highly educated and often feisty students. But the Genentech team was more than just a tough audience. They appeared to be intractable. As David recalls, the absolute futility of his quest became clear the moment the company's marketing person declared, "Well, if patients go blind in one eye, they still have the other. There's no market for this."

David was stunned. As an expert in the field, he knew that most patients' second eye would be affected within a few years.

CHANGING TUNES

Rejection was something for David to ponder as he flipped through the in-flight entertainment on the plane. Of all the movie stars and musicians listed on screen, who hadn't had their hopes dashed in their early days? Even the Beatles failed to impress the executives at Decca Records at the onset of their careers. No doubt Paul McCartney and John Lennon knew exactly how David felt at least once in their lives.

To be fair, Genentech wasn't the only pharmaceutical business seemingly stuck in the Jazz Age when David and his band of renegade eye-disease researchers were ready to rock. In many ways, the entire field of ophthalmology was dancing to its own drumbeat and never invited to the same party as other MDs. Compared to primary care physicians, heart surgeons, and bone specialists, eye doctors were oddballs. The level of commercial interest in ophthalmic drug therapies simply reflected this institutional prejudice.

As David's closest friend from his fellowship days at Harvard, Dr. Tony Adamis, explained many years later, "There was no formal ophthalmology training at medical school. It was a two-week elective, and, in the course's final exam, the final question on ophthalmology was 'How do you spell it?' That was the level of seriousness." Big Pharma reflected this oversight: The chief medical officers all tended to be oncologists or cardiologists with little to no introduction to ophthalmology in their medical education.

* * *

Back at the dawn of the 1990s, studying at Harvard, Tony and David were a pair of single guys outnumbered by classmates in relationships. They naturally fell into the rhythm of companionship, joining each other for dinner several times a week—as neither of them could cook—eating nachos at Division 16 or pasta and calamari at the Daily Catch. Tony was interested in the front of the eye and David, the back. Together they balanced one another, forming a fast friendship that has remained solid for the three decades since their fellowship.

Another important bond formed at Harvard was between David and Dr. Samir Patel. Samir was also deeply interested in retinal diseases. In Samir's case, this meant acquiring advanced surgical skills. He was drawn by the need for precision in the eye, doing everything under a microscope rather than slashing away using a big scalpel. Although David had a lot in common with both Samir and Tony, the three didn't coalesce as a group. Samir and Tony were aware of each other's presence in David's life, but their paths didn't cross very often during their fellowship years.

One day, while at Harvard, Tony attended a noon lecture, the kind where overworked med students typically nodded off when the lights dimmed. But this one, by a professor named Judah Folkman, awakened a deep passion. "I just was bolt upright in my seat taking notes," recalls Tony. "He was such a compelling speaker, and the subject matter was so interesting. I actually decided within twenty-four hours, I'm going to change my career. Instead of going back home and being a clinical ophthalmologist, I was just going to research blood vessels with this guy."

Known as the father of angiogenesis, Judah Folkman was a legendary figure in the war against cancer. In 1971, he laid out his visionary theory: For tumors to continue growing, they require the formation of new blood vessels—*angiogenesis*. He also discovered some of the fundamental biological mechanism behind this and what amounts to the process's on-and-off switch. However, these revolutionary findings were met with persistent dismissal by many in the medical research establishment. Also, unlike the prevailing medical research ethos, Folkman was interested in eyes, where the technical term for blood vessel growth is neovascularization. But it wasn't until the early 1990s that his approach of starving tumors of blood vessels, rather than simply killing malignant cells, was accepted by mainstream medical science and his lab began to develop clinical applications.

By that time, Folkman's lab had become the locus for innovative thinkers, like Tony, who were excited by the possibilities his discoveries opened. Folkman, the warm, modest son of a rabbi, embraced collaboration, and eventually, his thesis led to tens of thousands of academic papers, dozens of books, and numerous treatments for cancer and ophthalmic diseases. Orbiting around Folkman, at Harvard's Massachusetts Ear and Eye Infirmary and Boston's Children's Hospital, there was investigative work underway. But it was a discovery on the other side of the continent that propelled the next phase of angiogenic research.

Napoleone Ferrara, a molecular biologist from Sicily who gained his medical degree at the foot of fiery Mt. Etna and completed his postdoctoral research in the foggy precincts of the University of California, San Francisco, isolated vascular endothelial growth factor, a protein commonly referred to as VEGF. The protein had been uncovered several years earlier by Harold Dvorak and Don Senger at Harvard Medical School and labeled VPF (vascular permeability factor), but Napoleone's independent discovery in 1989 was rapidly followed by his sequencing and cloning of the molecule. VEGF's properties were not only understood, but with cloning, they became easier to study, and the name stuck. Clinicians had known for almost half a century that damaged retinas leaked something that could cause new blood vessels to grow in other parts of the eye. Over the years, this enigmatic material acquired the moniker Factor X. Now, thanks to Napoleone's discovery, Folkman and his acolytes quickly zeroed in on VEGF.

In a lab culture in 1992, Tony and his small team were able to grow retinal pigment epithelium (RPE), the compact single layer of cells that recycle the chemical debris thrown off by the photoreceptor cells as they absorb light and show that they produced VEGF. In other words, the eye could make its own VEGF. This was the first time ocular cells had been proven to do this. Importantly, this action was dependent on the level of oxygen deprivation. The lower the oxygen, the greater the production of VEGF. At the same time, Dr. Joan Miller, a member of the faculty at Massachusetts Ear and Eye who later became the chair of ophthalmology at Harvard, together with Tony, began conducting laboratory experiments. When retinas were damaged and lacked oxygen, they, too, created VEGF.

Determining the substance that promotes vessel growth in the retina is illuminating, but it didn't take too long to realize stopping VEGF was an important key to a successful therapy. Again, Napo, as Napoleone's friends call him, came to the fore. At the same time as Tony on the East Coast was showing the eye produced VEGF, Napo was able to produce an antibody that blocked VEGF in a living organism. Not only was Napo a brilliant scientist, but he also had the clarity of mind and drive to work at the one place in the world where his ambitions could be realized: Genentech.

* * *

Shortly after scientists first genetically engineered antibiotic-resistant bacteria in 1973, Herbert Boyer, a member of that scientific team, got a call from a young venture capitalist named Robert Swanson. In true Bay Area style, the pair met, agreed to invest five hundred dollars apiece, and launched Genentech, a name Boyer derived from *gen*etic *en*gineering *tech*nology and assembled in a manner linguistically paralleling the recombinant gene splicing that underpins the company's business model. They pioneered a revolutionary method for producing new drugs that involved cutting up DNA with enzymes, inserting foreign DNA, and then growing the altered combination in fermentation vats. The process was not only innovative, but it was also far cheaper than the traditional methods that relied on extraction from animals and plants.

The little start-up quickly proved its mettle by producing a human protein from *E. coli* bacteria. Within three years, Genentech was able to make human insulin using its recombinant process. Goodbye to insulin from pigs and cows. Hello to Wall Street! After this breakthrough, Genentech went public with a $35 million IPO in 1980 (roughly $135 million today). The ability to create and build recombinant antibodies at scale made experimentation much easier. In no time, the company became a global talent magnet. If you were the type of scientist drawn to molecular biology, like Napo, Genentech was where you wanted to be. In 1990, Roche bought a majority stake in Genentech for $2.1 billion. Nineteen years later, in 2009, Roche then acquired the remaining 40 percent of the company—which had more than amply proved its value—for $46.8 billion.

For anyone seeking anti-VEGF agents to conduct experiments, Napo's lab at Genentech was the only place to go. It was the source used by Tony and the team in Folkman's lab and the others around Boston. But by the time David knocked on its door, any trace of Genentech's humble origins appeared to have vanished. Now that Genentech was part of the larger pharmaceutical industry, it straddled a point of friction. Its "source material" science relies on openness, meaning ideas must first be shared to be reviewed by peers. But with billions of dollars at stake, commercialization fosters competitiveness. Once a scientific discovery is labeled as a company's "secret sauce," it's shared with those who have a seat at the table.

DOUBLE BLINDSIDED

Before David's disappointing trip to Genentech, its parent company, Roche, had already led him and his crew on a wild goose chase. Although to be fair, this was not at Roche's instigation. It was entirely the other way around.

In 1989, a San Franciscan ophthalmologist developed a special fondness for off-label use of one of Roche's oncology drugs: interferon-alfa-2a. Interferon, so named because it *interferes* with virus replication, was the first new anticancer drug created through genetic engineering in partnership with Genentech. It was initially approved for hairy cell leukemia—a spooky-sounding disease coined for the minute protrusions it causes on cancer cells—in 1986, and Dr. Wayne Fung inspired by Judah Folkman's work on interferon and its ability to treat tumors occurring in children's lungs and a particular cancer that forms in the lining of blood vessels showed promise for treating AMD. The amiable doctor tried it out in seven patients and claimed good results in six of them after a treatment program of regular injections that ran from six to eight weeks. Wayne Fung diligently explained all this in a letter to the *American Journal of Ophthalmology* in September 1991.

It's easy to understand Fung's enthusiasm. Curing blindness is what ophthalmologists devote their lives to, and the off-label use of prescription drugs is common practice by doctors of all sorts. Inspired by this apparent success, Fung and some other Bay Area eye doctors began to use interferon for AMD extensively. No stranger to the limelight, Fung, who was the personal ophthalmologist to the president of Taiwan in the 1980s, became their evangelist, spreading the good word at conferences and talking to the media.

Writing a considered letter to the *American Journal of Ophthalmology* is one thing; extoling the virtues of interferon for AMD in the pages of *USA Today* is another altogether. Interferon is far from an innocuous drug and comes with many side effects, most notably flu-like symptoms, nausea, and extreme tiredness, particularly when administered to older subjects, the core sufferers of AMD. Indeed, at the press conference heralding interferon's approval, FDA Commissioner Frank E. Young had sternly warned, "We advise caution in its use against other diseases . . . It would be premature to use it willy-nilly for any type of cancer." Without a doubt, given ophthalmology's orphan status in the pharmaceutical world, interferon's possible use for eye infirmities would have never even crossed the commissioner's mind. For the group of ophthalmologists orbiting Judah Folkman's lab, the lack of genuine research supporting Fung's claims was a vacuum waiting to be filled.

By that time, David was back in New York and had begun working at the highly esteemed practice of Lawrence "Larry" Yannuzzi, who, among many achievements, literally wrote the book about retinology. Together, Larry, Tony, David, Jason Slakter (another doctor), and Judah Folkman published an editorial in the October 1992 issue of the *Archives of Ophthalmology* (now *JAMA Ophthalmology*), questioning the "efficacy and safety" of using interferon-alfa to treat ocular diseases. Proof through properly orchestrated randomized clinical trials was urgently needed. Standard practices like using control groups, testing different dosages, and understanding treatment schedules on large numbers of subjects were of paramount concern.

Phone calls ensued. Roche began turning its wheels. Apparently, like all big drug companies, Roche was not well versed about ophthalmology. However, when David and Tony reached out to the pharma giant, they had the good fortune to get in touch with Judy Prestifilippo, who was remarkably enthusiastic about their line of inquiry. "After we met Judy," Tony explained, "we got invited to Basel, Switzerland, where we met Roche leadership, and we made the case that a proper Phase 3 trial needs to be done with interferon."

Quickly, David helped transform his group of friends into a team. They helped figure out what trials were needed to determine efficacy. "We designed it from scratch," Tony remembered. Together they would work with Roche, who would supply the drug, the funding, and what amounted to the general infrastructure of the trial.

Roche lacked a clinical trial leader who was an MD with expertise in ophthalmology. The tasks of crafting the study, setting it up, and training a team to run trials internationally fell into the lap of Denis O'Shaughnessy, an affable Irishman with a PhD in physiology...who was not so conveniently stationed in Strasbourg, France.

The research program consisted of two large, randomized studies of 500 patients each. In order to determine the correct dosage, each study population was divided evenly into four groups: 125 patients received a low dose, 125 received a medium dose, 125 received a high dose, and the remaining 125 formed the control group. For the participants, this meant receiving a dose consisting of either three, six, or nine units of medication every other day for a year. Adding to the complexity, the interferon, which the patients administered intravenously themselves, needed to be kept cold.

The full-blown trial spanned forty-five ophthalmic centers worldwide—from Helsinki to São Paulo and Tel Aviv—including nineteen locations across the US, which meant a lot of organization was required. Subjects were carefully vetted: Along with showing signs of AMD, each subject had to be at least fifty years old and without a heart condition, history of depression, major allergies, or any other adverse health condition. And not only did the dosages and drug delivery need to be standardized, so did the measurement of patient response, as well as the type and frequency of testing. Data collection, management, and analysis were other concerns. Plus, it was vital to monitor the safety of patients in case they had severe adverse reactions.

A RIOT IN VERSAILLES

Mobilizing an effort like this requires almost military precision. But in this case, the boots on the ground wear lab coats. Ophthalmologists, accustomed to running their own shows, make for rather restless troops. A year or so into the trial, to get everyone working in synchronicity, Denis organized a gathering in Versailles, France. It seemed like a good location. After all, far larger endeavors had been orchestrated from there in the past.

While Denis was en route to the big meeting, he received a call from Roche's head of global project management and portfolio management. Her news was not good. Roche was pulling the plug. As he recalls, he was told that "the portfolio couldn't accommodate it, and ophthalmology was not what Roche was interested in."

"I had a riot on my hands when I arrived at the meeting in Versailles," Denis said. The French and Italian delegations were calling for his head on a platter. Indeed, the leading French member and top French retina specialist at the time, Dr. Gabriel Coscas, "rejected" Roche's decision entirely, despite a lack of any means to do so. Fortunately, Evangelos Gragoudas, a Greek ophthalmologist and Harvard professor who completed his training in Boston, was also on the steering committee and convinced his European counterparts to "not shoot the messenger" and instead, focus on appealing to the powers that be.

After intense lobbying that went all the way to the top, Roche and the assembled ophthalmologists reached a deal. Instead of doing two studies, there would be just one, halving the number of patients needed. Also, the company would relinquish responsibility, handing over the New

Drug Application, the FDA's formal approval process, to David. Considering Roche made the drug, this was a highly unusual step, to say the least.

Consolidated in its new form, the trial went ahead. However, after a year, patients who received interferon did no better than those who didn't. In fact, those receiving the highest doses did slightly worse than the control group. The written report concluded that "interferon-alfa-2a provides no benefit as a treatment."

The entire exercise ended up costing Roche many millions of dollars. Not huge in the world of pharmaceuticals but still, at the time, an impressive sum to determine something is a dud. To the further detriment of Roche, the study revealed a new side effect not seen in the oncological trials, since eyes were the last thing on anyone's agenda. "Interferon-associated retinopathy," which causes small hemorrhages and fluffy white patches on the retina known as "cotton wool spots," needed to be added to the warning label on the drug. David thought this misadventure spelled the end—his first and final effort at bringing ophthalmology in line with other therapeutical research. He was very depressed. No doubt this was the end of his hope for a drug to fight AMD.

"Don't worry," Denis reassured David. "Nobody's ever run a big pharmaceutical study in retinal disease. And this is going to be the first of many." Rather than a door closing, Denis felt David had opened a window onto a whole new vista. He could set his sights on an array of drug companies eager to venture into ophthalmology. And, they were all going to call on David and Tony, since they ran the original study.

Now, as David flew back to New York, the long flight from the West Coast had given him time to ponder everything that had led up to the meeting with Genentech. He couldn't help but wonder about Denis's supposed silver lining. This whole global network he'd built to test ophthalmological drugs is precisely what he had just failed to sell to Genentech. Did it really have the value Denis assured him?

IT'S MARTY ON THE LINE

It turned out there was one person at Genentech with an acutely personal interest in eye disease. Marty Glick's mother had suffered from retinitis pigmentosa, a hereditary condition that left her legally blind from a young age. Then one day, during a business trip to New York, Marty's own sight became blurry. In no time at all, he lost all central vision in his right eye.

At first, Marty thought it had something to do with his contact lenses. His optometrist told him he had blood in his eye and needed to see a retinal specialist, pronto. It was quickly determined the problem in Marty's right eye was due to blood vessels in his retina leaking: He had myopic macular degeneration. This type of macular degeneration isn't related to aging; it targets people with high nearsightedness. Only in his forties, Marty heard the refrain familiar to the generation ahead of him: "There's nothing we can do." On the bright side, he was informed that the risk of it occurring in his left eye was very low.

Then, just two months later, his left eye started bleeding. But Marty refused to stop working. To cope with this sudden bout of legal blindness, Marty's staff blew up the font size of all his messages, at first to fifteen, then twenty, then thirty, and eventually forty points. He had people drive him everywhere. Despite his resolute productivity, with a wife and two kids, his life was completely nuts.

Marty asked around at Genentech, and, perhaps surprisingly, there was someone who knew quite a bit about eyes: an Australian researcher named Andrew Cuthbertson. Andrew self-deprecatingly describes himself as a "half-baked, stalled ophthalmologist," as he switched from studying ophthalmology to getting a PhD in molecular biology. But he acknowledges that he "definitely knew more about ophthalmology than anyone else at Genentech."

Aware of the research being conducted on interferon-alfa at that time, Andrew steered Marty to Wayne Fung. Convinced from what he'd seen with other patients, Fung signed Marty up under the experimental protocol and provided him with the drug.

Marty gave himself injections in his leg. And it seemed to work! His left eye calmed down, and his vision improved. With his contacts in, he was back to normal. "I was correctable with 20/20 vision with both eyes open," he remembered. Then, two weeks later, the bleeding returned. He called Wayne Fung and received another shot. The problem disappeared again. For Marty, the connection between interferon-alfa and macular degeneration couldn't have been clearer.

Marty wasn't a researcher or a marketer. He was a money guy. As Genentech's vice president of finance, he was second only to the CFO. Convinced firsthand of the potential of interferon for AMD, Marty ran through financial models for its possible market. The numbers sure added up. Interferon could be a billion-dollar drug!

When the negative results of the interferon trial came out, nobody was more baffled than Marty. To this day, he doubts his cure was simply a placebo effect and speculates interferon may work on a "certain genetic subsection" that he just randomly is a member of. However, retinal doctors would say that the myopic form of macular degeneration can get better by itself, unlike the age-related type, and stress that large, randomized controlled trials must determine if a drug actually works.

As colleagues united by their lonely belief in the necessity and value of developing a treatment for AMD, Marty and Andrew continued to talk. Their discussion moved on from Roche's interferon to the anti-VEGF work being done right down the hall at Genentech in Napo's lab. Andrew was also spellbound by Judah Folkman, whose work he knew from his student days and whom he had heard lecture at the National Institutes of Health (NIH), where Andrew was first employed in the US. He was convinced that anti-VEGF treatments could be extremely valuable for retinal diseases.

Napo had connected Andrew to Tony, Joan, and David, and they had become advisors to his research. It was through Andrew that David approached Genentech about using the company's anti-VEGF molecule to develop a drug for AMD. Naturally, Andrew was at the meeting that resulted in David's dismal departure.

Andrew related to Marty the story of David's disastrous exchange with the company's marketing executives that he witnessed unfold. Marty's experience with interferon didn't entail injections in the eye, but Andrew asserted that this wasn't a deal breaker despite what the marketing people said. Living in San Francisco through the early 1990s provided Andrew with a unique insight. AIDS was still at the height of its epidemic stage, and Andrew lived with his wife near the Castro district, the absolute epicenter of the disease. Afflicted gay men were coming down with all manner of infections due to their damaged immune systems, and cytomegalovirus (CMV), which can severely damage the retina and cause blindness, was rampant. Plenty of Andrew's neighbors underwent antiviral treatment for the condition, which required frequent injections directly into the eye—just like David's plan. When patients were given the choice between going blind or getting regular shots in the eyeball, the answer was obvious: Absolutely nobody backed away from the needle.

Besides, Andrew pointed out, delivering the drug directly to the affected area made it more effective and longer lasting. Plus, you needed less of it, making it more economical. (Music to a moneyman's ears.) Just as importantly, placing it in the eye cuts down on side effects in the rest of the body—you don't want nasty side effects elsewhere in the body. Andrew had even persuaded the uniquely talented protein engineers at Genentech to develop a special smaller version of their anti-VEGF molecule, which, in theory, improved its delivery in the eye.

GROUNDED. AGAIN.

Not long after David's flight landed in New York, his phone rang. Marty introduced himself. Could he come to New York to have dinner and discuss an alternative solution? In short order, Marty was on a plane. The two men met on the Upper East Side at Scalinatella, an Italian restaurant whose thirty-plus-year history makes it a culinary legend in a city renowned for its short-lived eateries.

Marty laid out his plan. He was going to circumvent the marketing people and directly approach Art Levison, Genentech's CEO. If Genentech wasn't prepared to go ahead with an ophthalmological drug itself, why not give it to David and let his team develop it? They could form a new company and take on the risk. However, being a Genentech employee, Marty couldn't run it. He suggested David could be the CEO. Marty and other board members would teach David business—a true learn-as-you-do street MBA!

When Marty eventually spoke to his boss, Levinson, a scientist himself, understood. After all, why let good research go to waste? And besides, who wanted to be in ophthalmology, anyway? He would bring it to the board for approval.

Finally, everything was falling in line. The next board meeting was coming up. David and his friends anxiously awaited the go-ahead.

But something unpredictable happened. Apparently, Herb Boyer showed up at the board meeting and he revealed he also occupied a seat on the board of Allergan, an eye care company. Resolute, Boyer may have torpedoed Art Levinson's plan and proposed giving the molecule to Allergan. Why would Genentech hand over something so valuable to a bunch of unknown newbies like this Guyer guy and his crew? A doctor who had never worked in the pharmaceutical industry, let alone run a company!

When David's phone finally rang, it wasn't at all what he had expected to hear. He was back to zero. With nothing on the horizon.

Chapter 2

THE BLUNT INSTRUMENT

Before Marty received interferon from Wayne Fung, he was presented with another option—laser treatment. Zapping people's retinas was the standard of care for macular degeneration in the 1990s after gaining traction in the previous decade.

In 1968, the year Apollo 8 became the first manned spacecraft to orbit the moon, sending back the iconic *Earthrise* photo on Christmas Eve and cementing the USA's lead in the space race, Dr. Francis L'Esperance, an ophthalmologist with a keen interest in astronomy, successfully used an argon laser for retinal vascular disease. Similar work was conducted by other pioneers like Dr. Arnall Patz and Dr. Charles Schepens. There's a poetic synchronicity between space exploration and the development of medical lasers; as the world turned its gaze skyward, the ophthalmic profession sought to shoot stars—or at least intense bursts of light—into our eyes.

For retinal diseases, this represented a giant leap forward from the medieval-sounding remedy of pituitary ablation. Prior to laser therapy, in the hope of decreasing the production of growth hormones, which influence the development of abnormal blood vessels, doctors would willfully destroy the "master gland" in the brain. Not only would patients lose a vital chunk of cerebral matter, but they would also need hormone replacements of all kinds for the rest of their lives—hardly a shining example of the Hippocratic oath's *primum non nocere*, Latin for "first, do no harm." Pituitary ablation was used on patients suffering from diabetic retinopathy rather than those with AMD, who, considering their likely lifespans, were simply left to go blind. Even so, it's little wonder in most cases doctors preferred to do nothing.

MAY THE FORCE BE WITH YOU

After almost two decades, the enthusiasm for lasers—to cut, vaporize, or congeal tissue—reached escape velocity. Call it the "*Star Wars* effect," the allure of lasers received a boost around the time Luke Skywalker started battling Darth Vader. What ophthalmologist wouldn't want to be seen as a swashbuckling medical wizard wielding the cutting edge of technology to banish blindness in a flash of light? Why not cauterize those pesky leaking vessels in the retina? Surely, with the precision now afforded by lasers, a treatment for AMD and diabetic retinopathy was finally at hand.

Photocoagulation—something that sounds like what happens if you spill your coffee on a magazine page—is the name for the procedure developed to stem macular degeneration and diabetic retinopathy (a similar condition caused by high blood sugar levels) with lasers. Despite the clunky moniker, photocoagulation became the hot topic at ophthalmological conferences around the world and quickly caught on among eye doctors. So much so that the need for a serious clinical study rapidly became apparent.

Diabetic retinopathy has remained the leading cause of blindness for people of working age in the US for the past fifty years and throughout the 1970s, and treating diabetic retinopathy with lasers was examined intensely by the National Eye Institute, part of the NIH. The Diabetic Retinopathy Study (DRS) aimed to find out if photocoagulation helped prevent severe visual loss and which of the competing types of lasers—argon or xenon—was more effective. By the middle of the decade, enough research had been done to answer one of those questions: Argon was victorious. For the remainder of the study, doctors were advised to use argon and later krypton laser—a piece of cautionary advice that was perhaps a portent of things to come.

By the end of the decade, when follow-up studies on patients were completed, a conclusion was reached: Laser therapy worked! In short, it didn't provide a cure, but it stopped deteriorating vision from getting worse. And it was definitely a step up from messing with patients' brains.

No sooner was the word out about laser's effect on diabetic retinopathy than the focus quickly shifted to macular degeneration. In 1982, the Macular Photocoagulation Study Group released its findings after observing patients aged fifty and older with vessel leakage away from the fovea, the area near the center of the macular responsible for seeing fine details and color. The study group's published results heralded good news: Compared to the disease's natural progression, after laser therapy, the risk of additional and severe loss of vision was reduced. The trial was stopped early. An anecdotal story was, apparently when asked before they were told the results, all but one principal investigator said, "Oh my God, it didn't work—we harmed people." Relying on their own eyes, the doctors simply didn't think it did any good due to the low level of efficacy that was hard to clinically detect. But there was nothing else at the time.

As a medical student, David thought the treatment was somewhat barbaric, akin to pituitary ablation for diabetic retinopathy. How could you destroy the very center of the retina with a destructive laser? It was the very part you wanted to save! Little did he know that his decision to do a fellowship at Harvard was to have more than academic consequences. Being in Boston would place him in the future home for drug treatment of retinal disease. However, when he began practicing back in New York, he had little choice but to toe the line.

For doctors routinely giving their elderly patients bleak news, laser therapy was the light at the end of the tunnel. And while drug companies steered clear of eyes, medical equipment manufacturers felt no such hesitation. Dimly lit eye doctors' offices have long been crammed with arcane apparatuses—hospital operating rooms even more so. In a very short time, laser treatment not only became widely accessible, but it also rose to the level of orthodoxy.

Even in their letter to the editor responding to Wayne Fung's interferon advocacy, David and Tony's group, along with Folkman, expressed caution: "We believe it is important to remind ophthalmologists of the guidelines of the Macular Photocoagulation Study Group relating to the appropriateness of prompt photocoagulation of treatable choroidal neovascularization." Such was the prevailing sentiment of the time. Laser, even though its efficacy was limited, was the standard of care, but only for some patients. The key word buried among the long scientific terms was *treatable*. Reading between the lines, this represented just a small group of macular degeneration sufferers, around 15 percent. And 50 percent would experience a recurrence of symptoms within six months of treatment.

Marty was a case in point. His right eye was too far gone. Shooting lasers at the center of his macular was unadvisable, as it destroyed the cells responsible for the most crucial aspect of a patient's vision. But Marty's left eye was a candidate. The bleeding he experienced was just off-center. Even so, the minuscule scar created by the laser could eventually expand, and he'd lose vision. It was this high level of risk that convinced him to opt for Wayne Fung's interferon shots instead.

Meanwhile, coming into focus was another school of laser treatment developed alongside photocoagulation: photodynamic therapy (PDT). In this drug-enhanced laser technique, a doctor first injects light-sensitive dye into a patient's arm, then, after placing a special contact lens on the patient's eye, the doctor shines a laser into the eye to activate the medicine collected in the retina. Upon activation, the medicine induces vessel closure. Unlike in photocoagulation, in PDT, the laser doesn't scar the back of the eye. Still, it ultimately proved to have limited efficacy and patient eligibility. But the medical advice Marty received at the time also discouraged him from going down this path, and considering the drugs that eventually accompanied the treatment weren't yet available, his reluctance seems particularly wise in retrospect.

Today, the gravitational pull of laser treatment for AMD looks like clutching at straws. But laser treatment's effectiveness was studied extensively. And while it did offer a temporary solution for some patients, the stabilization in vision was only minimal and could hardly be called a great treatment or cure.

Following the Macular Photocoagulation Study Group's first publicized results from randomized clinical trials in 1982, over the remainder of the decade, the group reviewed the long-term benefits of laser treatment. In 1991, it released an analysis of how much visual acuity patients treated with lasers had lost five years after treatment compared with untreated AMD sufferers. The conclusion was hardly stellar. They received minimal benefit. Perhaps even more disturbingly, in more than half—54 percent—of treated patients, bleeding reoccurred.

HINDSIGHT ISN'T 20/20

From our vantage point in the twenty-first century, it's easy to overlook the desperation of patients in preceding eras. From smallpox to HIV, the past is littered with diseases that once caused immense suffering but are now treatable or practically extinct; our collective memories of them have dimmed. This fading of familiarity with human frailty no doubt contributes to the rampant paranoia of today's medical skeptics. For AMD sufferers currently receiving anti-VEGF treatments, the prospect of only a short-term, barely halfway-decent outcome via laser therapy is not something readily considered, even if they could find a doctor who can still perform the procedure. There is little surviving evidence of the life they would have led just a mere generation ago. For better or worse, established medical cures are something we take for granted—even ones as life changing as the one David, Tony, Samir, and team were about to discover.

* * *

Although Henry Grunwald couldn't have realized it at the time, he had the profound foresight to document his visual decline caused by AMD and the way it affected his daily life. Grunwald died in 2005, on the cusp of the new era of drug treatment. His book, *Twilight: Losing Sight, Gaining Insight* (Knopf Publishers 1999), is a moving testament to the hardship that routinely affected millions. Following the development of anti-VEGF treatments, *Twilight* serves as a window into a bygone world. Best known for being the managing editor of *Time* magazine for two decades, followed by his stint as editor-in-chief of all Time, Inc. publications, Grunwald was one of David and Larry's patients. (It helped that David was in New York's premier retinal practice located on the city's tony Upper East Side.) Grunwald's journey into blindness began with a glass of water, which he failed to fill because he couldn't see it properly in a dimly lit room while on vacation in Italy. He blamed the hotelier for being cheap, saving on electricity with low-wattage bulbs. Back in the US, he visited Larry and David's office seeking a new prescription for glasses and learned the sad truth.

Grunwald's life in the media was built on reading text and understanding images; his "existence had been wrapped up in the printed word," as he describes it. Poignantly, the onset of the disease began after he finished serving as the US ambassador to his native Austria and just as he started working on his autobiography. In *Twilight*, he writes candidly about his descent into blindness.

"Macular degeneration did not condemn me to the equivalent of a polar night," Grunwald asserts. Instead of describing darkness, he painstakingly articulates the degrees of visual loss he experienced in tandem with the emotional effects and tremendous upheaval it caused his life and that of those around him. At the beginning of the book, he describes being at the beach: "The scene around me appears through a kind of curtain, a haze. If I bend down, I will have a hard time telling a stone apart from a shell, a coin from a piece of sea glass. If I were to pick up a discarded newspaper, I would not be able to read it."

Seeing objects in clear focus becomes impossible, and he finds it hard to distinguish colors. But the effect the disease has on his ability to communicate is particularly vexing. "Most of the time," Grunwald laments, "it is impossible for me to tell whether someone is smiling or frowning and whether a woman is pretty or not." Devastatingly, the truly intimate part of nonverbal conversation is eliminated. "Reading faces and the signals of mood and temper, which I had taken for granted as part of the art of seeing, has become extremely difficult except when I am inches away. Eye contact is nearly impossible."

His condition deeply impacted his social life: "I find that often I don't even recognize old friends and seem to cut them dead; at other times, I greet total strangers as old friends." The resulting confusion becomes a fundamental condition of existence. "One of the difficulties about macular degeneration is that those around you can never be sure what you see, and you yourself are not sure, either."

However, despite the deterioration at the center of his sight, his peripheral vision remained surprisingly intact, something that became clear when visited by his son, Peter: "He was surprised I did not notice that he had started to grow a beard. On the other hand, I was able to spot that one of his shoelaces had come undone."

Grunwald notes, "We receive 80 percent of our information through the eyes (or so the experts tell us)." Yet, the casual dependency built on top of visual perception to keep us informed is utterly demolished. "Scanning magazine headlines as I pass a newsstand, trying to find a name and floor on a building directory, deciphering labels in the medicine cabinet, glancing quickly through correspondence. Such fast sight bites are now usually beyond me."

For a man of words, this is particularly excruciating. "My greatest frustrations involve reading and writing," elaborates Grunwald. "After a lifetime during which these activities were as natural and necessary as breathing, I now feel the visual equivalent of struggling for breath."

Beyond causing frustration, Grunwald's condition plays havoc with his emotions. He faces unremitting depression, lapsing into "stretches of gloom and long silences." There are periods of denial, especially at the beginning of his descent, when his loss of independence is acutely disheartening. He writes about how many AMD sufferers pretend to go about their daily business unimpaired: "They continue to handle money without being able to see it clearly, stab at the wrong elevator buttons, and even drive cars far beyond the point of safety." He confesses, "I went through such a period." Even to the point of pretending to himself, he could read the newspaper when he couldn't. He quotes Dr. Josephine DeFini, a psychiatric social worker who was clinical director of social work and independent living services at the Lighthouse for the Blind, New York City, where over half of the patients suffered from macular degeneration: "Vision loss is like falling from the throne."

It's not surprising that facing such a dismal picture, AMD sufferers were particularly susceptible to clutching at false hopes. Grunwald recounts hearing Nick Stevenson—an affable World War II veteran who founded a support group, the Association for Macular Diseases—expound on this ill-founded optimism: "There is a strong tendency among us to go from doctor to doctor, hoping to find one who will say, 'Of course I understand; macular degeneration; here is what I'm going to do.'" But Stevenson was very clear: No doctor could ever say that.

Accepting the futility of the situation eventually led Grunwald to alter his behavior. "I noticed when someone was particularly careful walking down steps or when someone else was holding a menu very close to his eyes or looking at me in a somewhat vague, unfocused manner. Before long, I realized that these were signs of macular degeneration." These subtle actions were the response to the difficulty now posed by an array of daily activities. "Eating became a particular problem," Grunwald notes. In the dim illumination he endured in most dining venues, the food in front of him was "nearly indistinguishable." He would bite into a lemon believing it to be a shrimp or mistake bone for meat. Using a knife and fork was exasperating, like he had "entered a second childhood of messy eating." "Finding a saltshaker on a table is a major challenge," he continues, "and wine glasses are in danger of being upset by my uncertain hand." The effect of his newly developed clumsiness, he says, "reminded onlookers of a deep-sea diver laboriously reaching for scarcely visible objects."

His troubles didn't end at the dinner table. Smoking ceased to be an elegant repose, as he couldn't find the tip of his cigar to light or locate ashtrays. Grunwald's desk "became more chaotic than ever" as he lost sight of paper clips and scissors. Shopping was a bugbear, and there was no way to distinguish between items such as cameras, tape recorders, and radios. Today, those devices would be apps on his phone, but he would still have been unable to discern them. He writes about how the timeless New York pleasure of browsing store windows failed to enchant him: "A shop window full of shoes can look like a candy store and a cleaner can look like a deli." Even going to the bathroom could be hazardous, as he failed to decipher the hieroglyphs used for men's and women's restrooms. Additionally, stairs, curbs, rugs, and other low obstacles were ever-present dangers. In a city where jaywalking is practically a right, safety demanded crossing streets alongside fellow pedestrians, even using women with baby carriages as a form of armor.

Entertainment also lost its appeal. At the movies, sitting as close to the screen as possible, he found he was "apt to confuse the hero's face with the villain's." His apartment was filled with books, but instead of providing escape, his prized possessions demoralized him, as he was no longer able to read more than the cover. "The books mock me or thrust me into nostalgia," he notes.

One avenue that provided a glimmer of hope was technology, although not how we think of it today. A more apt phrase would be gadgetry. This was a rabbit hole that Grunwald gleefully bounded down, having always possessed a penchant for intriguing contraptions. He was "advised to try magnification" and "plunged into the realm of visual aids: magnifiers with built-in lights, reading lamps with lenses attached." Some of the reading aids he purchased bordered on sci-fi. He describes "a magnifying machine, which is essentially a closed-circuit TV set. A camera focuses on the text and blows it up on a screen." But despite its cutting-edge allure, he found using it tedious. "Even a short passage is frustrating, and the notion of reading a whole book that way overwhelms me. I think it would take almost as long as it would take those legendary monkeys to write *Hamlet*," he writes.

Grunwald learned of experimental products like the Low Vision Enhancement System being developed at Johns Hopkins University School of Medicine in collaboration with NASA. Perhaps a distant ancestor to Apple's Vision Pro but still in the Paleolithic era, it was "a kind of helmet with built-in TV cameras that enlarged the scene around the wearer." He notes, "With its power pack strapped on, it proved heavy and cumbersome, giving me the sensation of being in a diving outfit on dry land."

Mostly, the devices Grunwald encountered didn't deliver on their promises. But while he was busy scouring boutiques filled with large-lettered Monopoly and Scrabble games, researchers at venerable institutions like the Harkness Eye Institute at Columbia-Presbyterian (now known as the Columbia University Medical Center) were hoping to transplant healthy cells of the retina to replace damaged ones. At the same time, surgeons at Duke University and Johns Hopkins were trying their hand at new techniques, attempting to detach and rotate the retina to reposition the macula.

When these medical experiments caught Grunwald's attention, he asked his doctor about them. David's friend Samir had recently performed one of the first-ever transplants at the University of Chicago. In 1997, Samir told Grunwald's former publication, *Time* magazine, "It's an experiment. That's all it is."

"The good news," David elaborated for Grunwald's sake, "is that we are now able to surgically perform retinal transplantation, and there does not seem to be rejection by the eye of this foreign material. The bad news is that we still have no way to connect the approximately 1.2 million fibers from the retina to the brain. It's a nightmare with all that spaghetti in there."

In the end, Grunwald opted for the standard treatment of the time: laser therapy. Despite his reservations, with nothing else at hand, David administered it. Lasers made Grunwald nervous. He associated them with death rays from the science fiction of his youth. In a dark room with his head on a chin rest, held in place with a strap, he faced David across a familiar-looking eye examination machine that had a laser mounted on it. David's left hand pressed a tubular lens against Grunwald's right eye; in his right hand, David gripped a joystick, ready to beam a laser through the lens. After calmly admonishing his patient not to move, David zapped Grunwald's eye with a (temporarily) blinding flash. "Good . . . fine . . . very good," the doctor murmured before firing more beams at their tiny targets. Grunwald was unsure which of them—the patient or the practitioner—David was trying to reassure.

The procedure took all of three minutes. But Grunwald felt dazed for an hour. Later when Grunwald discussed the experience with his doctors, Dr. Yannuzzi told him confidently, "It's like splitting a diamond."

PLAYING HOOKY AT THE BEACH

Perhaps there was more to David's assurance during Grunwald's laser treatment than he realized. By the time he shot the abnormal vessels at the back of the retired editor's eye, David was keenly aware of the rising tide of discontent with laser treatment for AMD. Maybe subconsciously, David really did need to reaffirm his own belief that he was doing the best for his patient.

In his book, Grunwald used the beach as a metaphor for the increasing fogginess of his vision. For David and Tony, an unplanned visit to a beach several years prior had presented a moment of clarity. When the two East Coast friends were reunited at the American Academy of Ophthalmology's annual meeting in Anaheim in October 1991 (courtesy of their respective research departments), they decided to take advantage of Southern California's benign fall weather and head to the beach instead of the sunless conference hall. As science-oriented doctors, laser therapy's limitations had been gnawing at them since med school. It was something they needed to talk about freely. After all, what exactly was the value of a treatment that only helped a very small number of patients?

After the pair of young doctors slipped past the slender row of palm trees skirting Highway 1's concrete cordon and onto the bright sands of

Huntington Beach, the Pacific air unclouded their thinking. "I was almost brainwashed in a way as a student at Hopkins of how great laser was," David remembers. "That was the center for all the laser trials that showed laser worked." But he couldn't help but notice the limitations too: "Most people, 85 percent, were not eligible for laser; and of the 15 percent, half had recurred blood again in six months—and nobody got better vision." Despite all the lightsaber rattling, David's faith in lasers was never steadfast: "I'm saying to myself, 'Wow, they're all jumping up and down over something that doesn't really seem like it works that well.'"

As a surgeon, using lasers to repair detached retinas—a common condition often caused by aging, diabetes, or injury that needs immediate treatment—made sense to David. When eye surgeons "weld" a torn retina to the back of the eye, it's a precise operation with a high degree of success. But using it for AMD? David told Tony he felt, "more like an oncologist or a shrink." He continued, "You couldn't do anything. There has to be a better way. Laser is crazy."

Tony was similarly troubled. "It was the standard of care, but the average patient loses vision; they don't gain vision," he notes. His work in Folkman's lab was unveiling an alternative. "If the data were to translate to humans," he recalls, discussing against the backdrop of swaying palms, "drug therapy would be much more effective." Tony continues, aware that it's easier to make these statements from his present vantage point, "But back then that was very controversial. Do you go from lasers, which everybody knows and understands, to something we think would be a lot better?"

David had already encountered the kind of demoralizing institutional resistance that any advocate for change experiences. Just one year out of his fellowship, he was told by one of the biggest names in retina that his research into a drug for AMD would go nowhere—lasers were the solution! He remembers feeling terribly dejected after this chiding by a bigwig.

Of course, the pair of young ophthalmologists weren't the sole countervailing currents of thought outside the academy. As we've seen, farther up the Pacific coast, Wayne Fung was starting to make waves with his free-floating advocacy of interferon. And in the country's heartland, the fuzzy math of laser's efficacy was soon to be contested in what was fondly known as the "Great Retinal Debate" at an upcoming American Academy of Ophthalmology (AAO) meeting in Chicago.

The showdown was between two of the brightest leading lights in the ophthalmology universe. Howard Schatz was a retina specialist and clinical professor of ophthalmology at the University of California as well as director of the Retina Research Fund at St. Mary's Hospital and Medical Center—both in San Francisco. (Today, Schatz is world famous for his innovative photography. Shortly after the debate, he traded a stellar career of healing sight for an even more luminary one: providing the world with something to gaze upon by creating captivating images of dancers, boxers, models, and celebrities.) Schatz faced off against Lawrence Singerman, no neophyte himself. In 1977, Singerman founded the Macular Society, an international forum of investigators and clinicians devoted to retinal research, and among his numerous professional positions is director of retinal and laser surgery at Mount Sinai Medical Center, Cleveland, and principal investigator of the Macular Photocoagulation Studies (MPS) conducted by the NIH. Over his lengthy and distinguished career, Singerman has authored hundreds of papers and four books.

As Singerman recalls, he possessed the data. He showered the debate with studies that proved how lasers reduced vision loss, particularly the farther away from the fovea the treatment was applied. But ultimately, Schatz won the contest with an emotional appeal. Conceding defeat, Singerman relays how their battle ended. "Howard summed up, saying, 'If Mrs. Jones came to you, and you told her she needed laser based on the MPS, she would say, "If you treat me with laser, my sight will go down a lot immediately, and in three years it will only be slightly better than if I did nothing."'" Singerman vividly remembers Schatz concluded with this kicker from Mrs. Jones, "I get what's in it for you, but what's in it for me?"

For David, the debate encapsulated the problem: Laser damage can't be reversed. Grappling with the joystick in his office, he knew firsthand this was not what medicine was supposed to be about. Gradually he became determined to steer an entirely new course.

Chapter 3

A RISING STAR

While lasers were being used to treat people with AMD, preclinical work was underway deploying laser in other ways. This development was an offshoot and hopeful upgrade. In a remarkable twist, laser helped shine a spotlight on anti-VEGF treatments.

The laboratory work was in the hands of Joan Miller, now the chair of ophthalmology at Harvard Medical School. At the time, in the early 1990s, she was working at Massachusetts Ear and Eye and collaborating with Tony and Patricia D'Amore, a senior acolyte of Judah Folkman with a PhD in biology and presently the vice chair for Harvard's basic and translational research in the Department of Ophthalmology. Also on the team was D'Amore's graduate student David Shima, another biology PhD, who later became VP of ophthalmology at Roche. As mentioned earlier, it had been known for many years that damaged retinas secreted something that leaked into other parts of the eye, causing new blood vessel growth. One of those places was the iris. Joan and her colleagues were attempting to stop this growth with drugs developed by Judah Folkman, but so far none of them was working.

Joan and her team were also using parts of eyes to figure out what causes new blood vessel growth. Joan describes the experiments: "I used the laser to make an ischemic retina. . . . It would cause a protein to leak out and cause these abnormal new blood vessels to grow in the iris." A pattern emerged that looked familiar. Whenever oxygen was depleted, this mysterious substance—Factor X—that caused vessels to grow went up. It was the sequence seen in tumor growth. Joan and Tony's team was collaborating with Harold Dvorak, so the samples they collected were initially identified as VPF, but it didn't take long to realize that VPF and VEGF were one and the same.

The next step was using VEGF directly. Who had the VEGF they needed? Napoleone Ferrara at Genentech. Even though his focus was on cancer, he was happy to provide the ophthalmic researchers on the East Coast with what they needed. Joan and Tony found that VEGF injections made abnormal blood vessels grow. "It met all the tests," she recollects.

Now that Joan and her team understood the mechanism behind vessel growth, they could work toward their ultimate goal of stopping this process. Napoleone and Genentech again came to the rescue. "They gave us antibodies, and we were able to block the vessels in the laboratory model, so you could completely inhibit it," Joan explains. "It was way better than we expected." In the spring of 1995, Joan presented her data; the full VEGF story was clear to her: "This was the molecule you want to block. And Genentech had the antibodies. We had solved Factor X: VEGF was made in the retina and was associated with new blood vessel growth; and when you blocked VEGF the abnormal new blood vessels were stopped in their tracks."

Looking back at those early experiments, Joan acknowledges they also had limitations: "The science was harder to understand in macular degeneration, or at least harder to test because the laboratory models are not so good. We had far better science data on things more related to vein occlusion and diabetic retinopathy, what these preclinical models were better for."

ENOUGH PLAYING WITH MODELS

Down the corridor from Napoleone at Genentech, Andrew Cuthbertson was also aware of the unique challenge posed by AMD. "It was very hard to study because in diabetic retinal disease, the whole retina is ischemic; it's screaming out it needs more oxygen," Andrew notes. "You can put a needle in the eye and take a little sample, and you can measure VEGF in these patients because there's so much of it. The whole retina is making it." For AMD this isn't the case. "We couldn't detect it in the vitreous. It was too dilute," Andrew continues. By comparison, he explains, "Macular degeneration is a disease of the tiny sort—one-and-a-half square millimeters of the macula—and what's going on under that. So, it's impossible to get at." To prove his own VEGF hypothesis for wet AMD, he needed more than the preclinical data.

In Andrew's mind, panretinal photocoagulation for diabetic retinal disease had some justification, a sort of optical quid pro quo. "You would laser because there you would sacrifice the peripheral retina that was pouring out VEGF to save the macular," he explains. "But if the disease was in the macular or under the macular, how the hell do you do that?"

Fortunately, the enterprising scientist had imported an advanced research technique from his homeland. Developed at the Howard Florey Institute (now known as The Florey) in Melbourne, Australia, was a process called in situ hybridization. In Andrew's words, "It's a beautiful technique where you cut a microscope slide section of whatever you like—but in this case, human retina—and you make probes that will bind to gene products in the thing and then look at it under the microscope."

Andrew was able to get vitreoretinal surgeons in his network to send him specimens for his team to perform in situ hybridization on. "Real specimens," asserts Andrew, "where surgeons had gone in on patients who had the wet form of AMD, removed the blood vessels from under the macular, and sent me the specimens." He incubated the probes with the samples, so they bound with target cells and showed they were making VEGF. Despite the minuscule specimen size, Andrew's research provided a big piece of the puzzle. "So the VEGF *was* under the macula," he explains, "and we actually had evidence from human tissue."

Everything, all the research from both coasts, was pointing to the same conclusion. And to the same place. VEGF causes macular degeneration, and Genentech had the antibodies to block it. Andrew had even convinced Genentech's protein engineers to craft a smaller molecule, with only one of the usual two fragment antigen-binding (FAB) "arms" cleaved off so that it could be more easily deployed in the eye. "And we were able to show that, at least in preclinical models, it penetrated through the retina to the subretinal space, which is where the VEGF was," he states with a palpable enthusiasm that remains to this day. "It was such an exciting project. We were barreling along. Genentech was the only place I could get an anti-VEGF FAB fragment made to do my experiments. I mean, it was just magical." With the anti-VEGF FAB in hand, Joan and Tony showed that new blood vessels could be prevented form growing underneath the retina.

Everyone—Joan, Tony, Andrew, David, and all their research partners—agreed; it was time to do human trials. Tony, Samir, and David drafted a clinical program—an outline for how to conduct the trials. The recent experience with Roche's interferon provided a template. It was an exhilarating time. Finally, a treatment for AMD was at hand. All that was needed was to get it into people's eyes.

But higher up at Genentech, Andrew's excitement failed to be contagious. The focus was on cancer, for likely obvious commercial reasons. And at the meeting prior to David's disheartening flight back home, getting it into human eyes proved to be the sticking point. Despite millions of people going blind, apparently Genentech was in no rush. The senior ranks seemed to be more filled by commercial people, than with doctors, making decisions concerning medical issues. But even as financial leaders, there seemed to be a failure to see the market.

PLAN B?

Andrew decided to deflect the managerial snub by attempting to find partners who could perform the work Genentech wasn't prepared to do. Partnering with other companies that are more adept at some aspect of commercializing products in a particular medical field is common practice in the pharmaceutical industry. Getting a new drug to market is a very complex process, and often it's easier to piggyback off another firm's expertise—whether that's in research, licensing, manufacturing, or marketing. It can help spread the risk, speed things up, and reach new markets.

First, Andrew talked to Genentech's business people that he had relationships with: Marty Glick and John McLaughlin, the company's chief operating officer. He relayed the marketing team's failure to accept delivering the drug directly into people's eyeballs and convinced them this wasn't a problem. As Marty knew all too well, when you're going blind, you'll do anything.

But Marty and John would have to wait. Apparently, Genentech would not make ophthalmology a priority at this time. Cancer would come first. While Genentech was spinning its wheels, Andrew received an invitation from back home. "I got a call from an old medical school colleague, Brian McNamee, the thirty-three-year-old CEO of CSL," he explains. An Australian company formed to produce vaccines during the adolescent nation's isolation in World War I, CSL, originally called Commonwealth Serum Laboratories, had recently been floated on the Australian Stock Exchange and was poised for a larger role on the global pharma stage. The young CEO made an offer too good to refuse: "Why don't you come back to Australia as head of research?" For Andrew, it was the only job in Australia that could compare to what he was doing in San Francisco. And seeing as what he was doing in San Francisco was at a dead end, he had no hesitation about moving back across the Pacific.

HUNTING FOR A MOLECULE

With Andrew gone and the front door and side doors firmly closed at Genentech, the back channel opened by Marty was still in play. His overture to David to run a biotech company with his and John McLaughlin's part-time assistance stood firm. But lacking Genentech's anti-VEGF molecule to put into human trials meant their undertaking remained rather abstract. You can't conduct human trials with just an idea. Still, it wasn't as though David was left idle. His clinical work at Yannuzzi's practice continued at its usual pace, and he had the ophthalmology program to run. Indeed, having one foot planted in academia was a huge advantage.

It meant David was always abreast of the latest developments in science. Research doesn't occur in a vacuum. Once the principle of VEGF causing angiogenesis was established and Napoleone's antibodies understood, the broader research community first reproduced the experiments and then began to build upon them in other ways. One such development was VEGF-Trap, a drug developed by Regeneron Pharmaceuticals, which eventually became known by the brand name Eylea. A recombinant fusion protein, it acts as a "trap" by binding to VEGF and stopping it from interacting with the receptors on cells' surfaces. This way, it interrupts the signals that otherwise would stimulate new blood vessel growth.

In the latter part of the nineties, VEGF-Trap got on David and Tony's radar. They arranged to meet with Regeneron's founders, Len Schleifer and George Yancopoulos. The company began when Schleifer, inspired by Genentech, spotted a gap in the market for research on diseases of the nervous system—hence the name Regeneron, derived from *regenerating neurons.* After some initial difficulties—including a failed attempt to treat Lou Gehrig's disease—the company's focus switched to diseases with better understood biological profiles that allowed for faster development, prompting its interest in VEGF.

When Tony and David went to present to Regeneron's board, they were surprised to discover that out of the ten people in the room, four of them were Nobel laureates. Tony, despite having given dozens of lectures around the world, had never been more nervous than he was in front of this small, select group. David recalls that these intellectual powerhouses took no time to get up to speed: "They were so smart. Within three minutes the Nobel laureates turned out to be masters of ophthalmology, even though they initially knew nothing about it."

But just prior to the meeting, David learned that even the world's most revered intellectuals have their limitations. Before the start of proceedings, one of the laureates was trying but failing to get coffee out of a complicated urn. Never one to let anything disrupt his access to caffeine, David offered to help. "So, I come and I say, 'Oh, let me show you how.'" David recalls as he carefully demonstrated how to fill a cup. "I get him his coffee, and he looks at me and says, 'You are a genius!'" Not only did this declaration make David's day; it also set up his evening, too. Later that night, he was able to impress his date: "I said, my friend and I lectured in front of four Nobel laureates, and one of them said I was a genius."

Similarly, Yancopoulos and Schleifer were impressed by David and Tony's compelling argument to license VEGF-Trap for use against AMD and by its clear market potential. But unfortunately, their hands were tied. At that moment, VEGF-Trap was snared in a joint venture with Procter & Gamble, who had no desire to use it for the eye either through in-house development or licensing. It was the same old story from Big Pharma about ophthalmological drugs but this time wrapped in an innovative new package. At a recent Eyecelerator gathering, a forum for ophthalmic innovation, Schleifer and Yancopoulos said that if they had gone with David and Tony, they would have developed Eylea ten years earlier.

Given the importance of their mission, David and Tony were constantly on the lookout for possible partnerships and licensing arrangements. But for once, they were on the receiving end of an inquiry. Inspired by Tony's paper on increased VEGF levels in eyes with proliferative diabetic retinopathy (which included research from Joan, Folkman, and others), Nebojsa Janjic, a scientist at a small company far removed from the familiar centers of biotechnology in Boulder, Colorado, reached out to them. Nebojsa had decided a molecule he was working on for cancer might, in fact, be better suited for eye disease. He approached Tony and David to see if they would act as consultants.

Nebojsa was working with an *aptamer*, a new type of drug consisting of a synthetically developed single strand of nucleic acid that works in a similar manner to antibodies. To create an aptamer, an extensive collection of either random DNA or RNA sequences is exposed to a target molecule. The ones that bind to the target are chosen. Additional rounds of selection increase the affinity and narrow the array of possible aptamers. Eventually, one is optimized and stabilized for use. When deployed, aptamers can inhibit protein-to-protein interactions or send enzymes, proteins, and other particles and agents to specific cells or tissues. They are extremely accurate in their targeting, which reduces the risk of unwanted effects.

Originally, the anti-VEGF aptamer Nebojsa developed was tested on laboratory tumor models. After learning about Tony's work, maybe, Nebojsa conjectured, it would perform better if injected directly into the eyes.

Nebojsa was working at NeXstar, a relatively new company focused on aptamer development founded by serial entrepreneur Larry Gold, who was a professor at the University of Colorado. Gold went on to be elected to the National Academy of Sciences, but at the time Nebojsa contacted David and Tony, the work at NeXstar warranted deeper investigation. So David, Tony, and Marty, who was still a VP at Genentech, went to Colorado to get a better understanding of how they could benefit from this new technology and the aptamer in question.

Tony validated the aptamer's anti-VEGF science, and David reviewed the clinical studies behind it. Nebojsa's hunch was a good one. Marty evaluated the potential. "The reality was there was nothing going on," Marty recalls about the state of the market. "The big guys—Alcon, Allergan, Bausch & Lomb—were quite honestly sleepy companies not doing any breakthrough retinal research. They're working on their niche products." Clearly, NeXstar had zero experience with ophthalmology. But if David and Tony got the aptamer, they'd be in the clear. Introducing a groundbreaking treatment for AMD was a golden opportunity, and Marty felt he could raise the money to back them.

"The whole point was," Marty recounts, "if we do this, we have to take control. It's going to be our baby." And he got to work. He had a lot of talks with NeXstar. Then he approached bankers and discussed financing.

Momentum began to build. He felt it was a go with NeXstar. "We had a handshake deal," he recalls. "And so, I took a deep breath and resigned from Genentech." After ten and a half years at Genentech, Marty didn't take the decision lightly. Particularly as it meant kissing goodbye to a large pile of stock options.

DATING EXPIRATION

Around the same time Marty was getting ready for a major upheaval, David's personal life was changing direction. Instead of saying farewell to expectations, David was embracing a whole new set of possibilities.

A woman David knew, Maria Marino, had gradually, over the course of years, transformed from a friend of a friend to a close friend to a girlfriend. "When I learned David had connected with Maria, at first, he just sounded different," remembers Tony of his former Boston bachelor buddy. "It sounded like she was the one, and it's been borne out by time. They're still together and very happy."

The pair met when David, as an up-and-coming ophthalmologist, followed the great tradition of New York intelligentsia, from the abstract expressionists to John Steinbeck and Truman Capote, and got a share in the Hamptons, a seasonal rental where a small group of like minds could relax and mingle while escaping summer in the city. Maria, invited by one of David's companions, didn't struggle to make an impression.

Having grown up in the Boston area, Maria quickly found her feet on arrival in New York, working for the musician Sting before landing a gig at MTV Network's VH1 as it transformed from a video jukebox into a global culture powerhouse. Working in this communication crucible allowed Maria to experiment as an on-camera personality and off-screen producer. She was open to ideas, including one from David about reporting on the music doctors liked to listen to while performing operations. After VH1, Maria moved on to other media outlets, including Metro TV where her on-air reporting, in pursuit of authenticity, included jumping out of planes. Eventually, by the time she and David were ready to explore living together, Maria had settled into a more predictable producer's path at A&E.

Not long after David and Maria joined forces, the time came for Tony, David, and Marty to sit down again with NeXstar. The trio went back to Colorado. But instead of signing on the dotted line, NeXstar had a change of heart. Rather than hand over the aptamer, they wanted to keep control. "Basically," reflects Marty, "they reneged on doing the deal."

To say the air went out of the bag is an understatement. How could Marty finance a company without a potential product in the pipeline? The team continued to look around for alternatives. Nothing in the anti-VEGF space rose to a level that warranted pursuit.

David continued his clinical and academic work, and Tony stayed busy in the laboratory. Eventually, Marty had to take a job. He wound up at Theravance, a publicly traded biopharma company, as executive vice president and CFO.

Then one day, while Marty was sitting at his desk at Theravance, something in the newspaper caught his eye—a story about NeXstar. Gilead Sciences was set to acquire it. *Just maybe, that aptamer would be up for grabs after all...*

Chapter 4

A BALM IN GILEAD

"Hey, I'm the CFO at Theravance. I was once at Genentech. I know a lot about this drug." Marty was on the phone, a cold call with his counterpart at Gilead, John Milligan, then head of business development and future CEO, whom he'd never met. "Would you consider spinning it off to a small company?"

The small company Marty referred to wasn't Theravance. It didn't have a name or an address or really even exist—yet. But that didn't stop Marty from sensing an opportunity and acting on it. Following the announcement of Gilead's acquisition of NeXstar, the bigger story started to spill into the news. Gilead was going to focus on antivirals, particularly for AIDS. Marty knew Gilead had no ophthalmology experience, and it was clear they weren't about to develop any. When Gilead made its desire to spin off noncore assets public, it meant NeXstar's aptamer was up for grabs.

After creating Tamiflu, the widely used antiviral medication for influenza A and B which had just received approval, Gilead was forced to license it to Roche to complete its development and go to market. This was not an exercise John Martin, Gilead's CEO, wished to repeat. The acquisition not only gave Gilead access to AmBisome, an antifungal treatment, and two AIDS drugs, DaunoXome and Vistide, but it also brought on board NeXstar's international salesforce, saving Gilead the time and trouble of developing its own. In many ways, the acquisition was a means for Gilead to leapfrog a few steps up the pharma food chain.

Whatever its motive, Gilead's move signaled it was building momentum. This meant there was no time to waste. Marty reached out to David and Tony. "Let's dust off this idea again. I still want to do it," Marty recalls saying. But there was just one problem. He had a full-time job. "So, I asked David, 'If we do this, can we base it in New York? And you be the CEO?'" David, who had not one but two jobs and had never run a company before, answered yes.

Even though David lacked business experience, it wasn't as if they were starting from scratch. In the run-up to the previous attempt to get the aptamer, they had put together a top-notch business plan. They had all the original modeling based on existing market data as a foundation. Then, they created an investor pitch. The conclusion was clear: For a completely unmet medical need based on a chronic condition—one likely to require patients undergo treatment for another ten to fifteen years—this was a multi-billion dollar drug.

David's first task was to reactivate the team he'd assembled for the interferon trial. It wasn't the only time he'd done this. Shortly after the trial, Roche decided to wind down its Strasbourg office, and Denis O'Shaughnessy, who had told David that despite the trial's failure it was a key to the future, opted to relocate to Roche's US headquarters in New Jersey, putting him in close proximity to David. Denis was skeptical when he received David's call. "I used to get phone calls from David with a potential opportunity of forming a drug company around Christmastime each year," he recalls. From the previous false starts, Denis had already assembled a clinical plan using the experience with the interferon trial, including its global network of ophthalmologists, to recruit patients. As ophthalmology was such an outlier, no one else could claim to possess a plan. But this time, David wasn't crying wolf. Milligan had responded positively to Marty's overture. There was a meeting scheduled at Gilead's headquarters in Foster City, halfway between San Francisco and Silicon Valley.

Companies are built of two things: talent and money. Given that this new company led by David entirely lacked the second component, it was vital to impress the Gilead folks with the former. Technically, no one attending the meeting was an employee of the phantom company. But that was a minor detail. They were all employed somewhere, armed with an impressive array of skills and performing at the top of their games. The fact that they could all assemble in the same place on the West Coast at the same time with little advanced notice was evidence they functioned as a well-oiled team.

On the financial front, Marty from Theravance was joined by John McLaughlin, who, after years in senior management and COO at Genentech, was currently president of Tularik, a biotech start-up later bought by Amgen for $1.3 billion. Together they presented a formidable force of pharma business acumen. The trio of doctors—David, Samir from the University of Chicago, and Tony from Harvard—clearly showed the underlying science was understood. Even though he was firmly on Roche's payroll, Denis brought his expertise in running clinical trials to the table. Rounding out the bench was Harsha Murthy, a pro bono lawyer, ready to weigh in firsthand on any legal developments.

The meeting with Gilead's top brass went surprisingly smoothly. To his credit, John Martin, Gilead's CEO, recognized the potential and could see the value in handing over the aptamer to an organization led by eye doctors. Given the usual treatment ophthalmology experienced at drug companies, Martin's response was nothing short of heroic. After the meeting with the full team, Martin and Mulligan pulled Marty, David, and John aside to hash out the financials. Everything was set to go. A celebratory dinner was in order.

A CLOSE CALL

To accommodate the assembled teams, the dinner was held in a large nondescript restaurant in Palo Alto. It was not the cozy kind of place where you'd expect to run into acquaintances, particularly not if you were from the other side of the continent, much less the planet. But when Denis responded to the call of nature, that's exactly what happened.

"I got up to go to the bathroom, and I saw my boss from Europe walking in," Denis remembers, the awkward occasion stuck in his memory. "It was too late to turn around. I just had to keep walking. And then we ended up in the toilets together."

His boss, although based in Basel, Switzerland, was, for some reason, in California—at that very moment. Alongside each other at the stalls, they both had the same thought cross their minds. "And he said, 'What are you doing here?'" Denis remembers. He then made a quick calculation. He didn't think his boss had seen him at the table with John Martin. It would be very difficult to explain why he was having dinner with the CEO of a rival drug company, especially one that was getting press attention. The old proverb, discretion is the better part of valor, took hold, and Denis got creative: "I'm on vacation visiting family who live out here." He hoped his boss wouldn't pry. "I thought, please don't start in asking me about where they live and all the rest of it." Fortunately, his boss left it at that.

When Denis returned to the table, his companions thought he'd seen a ghost. A religious man, Denis felt this visitation signified something. What exactly, he wasn't yet sure. Although one thing Denis was certain about was that he had no intention of leaving Roche to work for a start-up, not at his age, having turned fifty with two kids in school. If nothing else, seeing his boss confirmed that. This jaunt was way too risky.

THE GOLDEN HANDSHAKE

By the end of the meal, the future of the aptamer had been sealed. John Martin was confident it was going into good hands. Ophthalmology drugs should be under the watchful care of ophthalmologists. After all, who else knew anything about eyes? If there was a reason why eye diseases stayed off the radar of Big Pharma, it wasn't Gilead's mission to find out the hard way.

But there was just one more thing. Money.

David had proven they had the skill sets on hand to do the necessary research for the aptamer to be approved. However, the aptamer wasn't a gift. It was an asset, one with potentially a lot of value, as Marty's calculations revealed. And even though this new small company was the ideal recipient of the molecule, it wasn't the only entity inquiring about it.

If Marty, Samir, Tony, John, and David wanted the aptamer, they had to beat the competition. John Martin set a time limit. They had twelve days to raise $8 million or else lose their spot at the head of the line. After almost half a decade of lost opportunities, things were about to get real. And fast.

Chapter 5

THE RACE IS ON!

Long before everyone began staring at their smartphones, medical professionals (when on call) carried pagers. But at the dawn of the twenty-first century, when John Martin launched his call to action, the Blackberry had just hit the scene, uniting email with voice. What now looks like a clunky marriage of mechanization and high tech was the sleekest new tool for doctors about to become businessmen overnight. No sooner had the funding countdown commenced than Samir Patel reached for his Blackberry—and put his network on call.

Today, we think of an influencer as someone who, by raising the palm of their hand, reaches millions of people instantly. Samir, however, was a different type of influencer, someone who only needed to reach handfuls of people to raise millions. Most of those people were also Patels—a community who trace their origins to Gujarat in India. In Samir's case, a journey that crosses four continents.

Samir comes from a family of doctors. His father was a physiatrist who provided medical oversight to diagnostic and rehabilitation services alongside a group of neurosurgeons. Neurosurgery was a career that Samir also considered, which is why it's no coincidence that after being attracted to ophthalmology, Samir's focus was the part of the eye that sends signals to the brain. Samir's uncle and aunt were also doctors, but Samir's familiarity with ophthalmology stems from a different, unfortunate familial connection. Shortly after arriving in the US, on her high school graduation day, his older sister was struck in the eye by a firework. Living in central Massachusetts at the time, she had to go to the Eye and

Ear hospital in Boston daily for treatment. Samir, then thirteen years old, would accompany her, and the ongoing care for her severe injury had a lasting impact on the young, aspiring doctor. It created an appreciation for an often obscure medical field.

So when the time came to raise money for a potential blindness treatment, Samir knew his wider family circle would likely be sympathetic to the urgent need for funds. Enabled by his BlackBerry, Samir quickly sifted through, then contacted family and friends who possessed the means to help and an understanding of the medical necessity behind their investment. He swiftly coordinated conference calls, emailed documentation, and answered questions. Luckily, it wasn't the first time he'd done this. While training as an intern, he'd also solicited financing. Back then, his target audience—mostly fellow medical residents in his cohort—was also close at hand (though not so financially well endowed). But there was nothing medicinal about this first investment opportunity; it was for a unique real estate opportunity—one that only could exist in Chicago.

* * *

While finishing his training in Chicago, it came to Samir's attention that a mere sixty blocks from the Loop, land was selling for just three dollars per square foot. Quite a bargain. But there was a reason for this extreme discount. The territory was gang and drug infested. However, this didn't trouble Samir in the least. Venturing onto the turf in his Lincoln Navigator, he felt a measure of respect from the locals. After all, only certain types of people would be so bold, and prospecting doctors didn't come to mind.

On foot, Samir came across people lying in stairwells and other signs of urban squalor, but it failed to unsettle him, as this was nothing compared to his childhood. Growing up in turbulent times in East Africa meant regularly witnessing the kind of violence where people lost limbs to machetes. Being in a medical family brought this trauma extremely close to home—a home that was forever lost, when his family was expelled from East Africa by the dictator Idi Amin, along with about eighty thousand other people of South Asian descent. His family was given just ninety days to pack up and go, allowed to take only a minimum of possessions, and forced to surrender their business and landholdings in a violent attempt to redress perceived distortions in the East African economic system, instigated by the British during colonization. For Samir, it led to a short period as a refugee in India, followed by a stay in the UK.

His residency as a guest of Her Majesty's in the UK bore a strong resemblance to the terrain Samir surveyed in Chicago. While reacquiring his medical accreditations to practice in the country, Samir's father found employment administering electroshock therapy at a mental institution in a dismal postindustrial estate in the hinterlands of Glasgow. Samir experienced firsthand the kind of bleakness that leads to drug abuse and despair in cities in the Western world. Having survived so much himself, Samir was also capable of envisaging a different future. At a rock-bottom price per square foot, any improvement would likely lead to a return.

After successfully convincing his colleagues and friends to invest in the land venture, they didn't have to wait long to be rewarded. The city of Chicago stepped in to claim the land under eminent domain. While this undermined any long-term vision Samir and his investors may have held, the nine dollars per square foot paid by the government was a very solid 300 percent profit. The young doctor may have lost a tract of land, but he established a track record of knowing a sound investment when he saw one.

* * *

Connected to a tightly woven community with a deep appreciation for both opportunity and sacrifice, Samir was able to quickly rally his relatives and friends to secure a significant amount of financing for this new venture, called Eyetech. It wasn't difficult for them to conceive of the value and potential of Gilead's aptamer, despite both its complex nature and the lack of precedent in ophthalmology drugs. At the end of his efforts, Samir managed to get twenty-two Patels to commit. Included in this group was a friend, Tom Elden, with a family office, a private wealth management firm that handles investment and financial planning. Having a wealth management firm on board represented a step-up in fundraising, adding considerably to the coffers and, most importantly, to the effort's credibility. Once professional wealth managers see value in an investment, maybe it really *is* legitimate. When that investment has attracted $8 million virtually overnight—the sum Samir raised—not only is it legitimate, but it's also worth looking into.

A STAMPEDE OF WET FEET

Investors like to boast about when they "got in early and rode the wave to its peak." But the truth is, almost no investor wants to be the first to put their toe in the water. Even those with a "high risk tolerance" usually don't like to take on all the risk themselves. They'd rather share it; consider this capitalism at its most benevolent. And the simplest way to ensure risk is divvied up is by being the second or third to dive in. That way, you know you're not alone, hoping someone will throw you a lifeline if things go wrong.

Samir's rapid capital raising had a quick knock-on effect. If all these Patels were so keen to invest, perhaps there was something to it after all. Eyetech was now more than an idea. The Patels' backing made it real. The aptamer was secured. Someone—a group of high-net-worth individuals plus a family office—was willing to take on the risk. From here on, every investor added diluted the risk.

The required $8 million upfront was now in place, but more funds would be needed over the long term. Gilead's licensing deal required another $30 million to be paid over time at various milestones, such as $5 million when the New Drug Application is filed in the US, and $3 million when it's filed in the EU. Then other sums were due when sales began in different regions; plus there were ongoing royalties starting at 10 percent of net sales worldwide and increasing in the US as sales volumes went up. In short, Samir's lightning effort signaled the beginning of a larger money-raising endeavor.

Likewise, Marty didn't lose any time soliciting funds after John Martin's imperative; it just added to his prodigious workload of eighty to ninety hours per week. Theravance was aware of this and didn't mind. He was the kind of guy who gets things done.

* * *

A friend of Marty's at Merrill Lynch introduced him to Hingge Hsu. Hsu was a doctor, receiving his MD from Yale Medical School, but he was also a businessman—and not one who learned business on the fly. He was fully fledged, with nothing less than an MBA from Harvard Business School. When Hingge showed up on the West Coast in Marty's office at Theravance, he was a partner at Schroder Ventures Life Sciences (now SV Life Sciences), the Boston-based venture capital fund that began the year before with a pot of $310 million.

Aside from credentials, experience, and deep pockets, Hingge also possessed a key attribute: imagination. Before the meeting took place, no venture fund had ever invested heavily in drugs for ophthalmology. It was considered a field devoid of opportunity, except for the lucrative market in ophthalmic medical devices. Most forecasting—from weather to financial modeling—relies on projecting past patterns into the future, with a little tweaking here and there depending on the variables. When there is no past, how can you predict a future outcome? As Marty explains about typical investors, "they looked in the rearview mirror, and all the drugs in the ophthalmic market were small. And so instead of looking forward to an opportunity, they looked backwards." But not so Dr. Hsu.

Hingge's unusual powers of imagination were on full display when he met David, who had flown to San Francisco at Marty's behest. The three men gathered at a restaurant for breakfast. David was without his usual stack of presentation slides and instead resorted to old-school visualization: putting pen to napkin and literally sketching out the pitch. From this napkin blueprint, Hingge immediately grasped the full potential, the multi-billion dollar opportunity. And he told Marty, "I'm willing to fund it." Less than a month after John Martin agreed to license the aptamer, Eyetech was a $40 million company.

With VC money now behind it, Eyetech was in play. It could fund a drug trial. But first, the start-up had to actually get going. Although launching in an ocean full of start-ups who were busy burning venture capital, it wasn't long before this little company started making big waves.

EYETECH IS NOT A DOT-COM

In early 2000, the dot-com bubble was at its point of maximum inflation. A torrent of tech companies bought Super Bowl ads, including the infamous Pets.com, its sock puppet mascot epitomizing the illusion of hype. The NASDAQ reached its peak of 5,132.52 during the trading day of March 10. That was roughly double the index's value of the year before and a 400 percent increase from the mid-nineties. The price-to-earnings ratio of 200 was nothing short of surreal. (For reference, the S&P 500 generally has a P/E ratio of around 20.) Quitting your job to day-trade became a smart career move while expecting companies to turn profits was suddenly seen as passé.

The name Eyetech captured the flavor of the moment, a sleek way to signal the company's forward-thinking approach to tackling eye disease. It represents Eyetech as an industry disruptor and evokes a penumbral sentiment of the soon-to-be-eclipsed era of lasers. Although the company was squarely focused on therapeutics, the name was redolent of medical devices, forming a bridge to the coming era. Like for so many companies of the moment, the challenge for Eyetech was turning an idea into a reality. But Eyetech had one key point of differentiation: The core of its business model was a molecule, something tangible, not just an arrangement of ones and zeros.

The first order of business for Eyetech was turning their investment into a drug trial. Before you can start a trial, you need to establish the protocol, the road map for researchers, sponsors, regulatory agencies, and participants. David immediately turned to Denis, and Denis turned to someone at Roche he could trust, Evelyn Harrison. Evelyn was aware of Denis's work with the interferon trial; she wasn't involved, but they worked together on other projects and had a solid relationship.

Evelyn earned her undergraduate degree in biology, then worked as a research assistant at Cornell University's medical school for almost five years in the Division of Infectious Diseases, ultimately running a lab studying cryptosporidiosis for HIV patients. When Pfizer and Roche both offered her jobs, she opted for Roche. As a single African-American woman in her late twenties, Groton, Connecticut—where Pfizer's research and development labs were located—had zero appeal. "[Choosing Roche], she later said, "was the best decision of my life."

Over dinner with David at a small restaurant on the Upper East Side, she learned about him acquiring the drug and the company he was starting. When she asked where the company's office was, David had to tell her he didn't have one. David was a fast talker, but she was won over by him. He was passionate and convincing, and clearly, the need was enormous. Setting up a trial for this new AMD drug was definitely worth considering. She would mull it over.

Having spent almost ten years at Roche, one of the world's biggest pharma companies with thousands and thousands of employees around the globe, Evelyn felt hesitation. "This sounds great in theory," she remembers thinking, "but I don't know. How is he supposed to do this as a one-man show? Has he stored the drug in his refrigerator?" She confided her reservations to Denis. And he felt similar. However, the pair had no issues working with David as consultants. Who doesn't like to make a little extra money?

For the time being, that was fine with David. He was looking for a place to house full-time employees but hadn't signed a lease yet. Plus, as a brand-new businessman running a brand-new business, there were plenty of other details requiring his attention.

Evelyn needed assistance getting David's protocols in order; after all, she had just stepped up a few rungs on the ladder at Roche, being promoted to director of virology, with a full portfolio of studies to oversee. Luckily, her former administrative assistant Lillian Vasquez was at a loose end and needed a gig.

When Evelyn was starting at Roche, they began working together as part of a program that trained high school students and gave them jobs. Lillian was familiar with all the clinical research needs for the protocol. But not long before Evelyn reached out, Lillian had grown tired of Roche and went to work at a bank—a move that didn't pan out. When Evelyn talked to Lillian about Eyetech and asked if she'd consider getting involved, a meeting with David was arranged. Lillian liked David but was a little spooked by the complete lack of anything resembling a bona fide company—like, for example, an office.

Evelyn arranged for Lillian to work at her house in Denville, New Jersey, an hour north of the Pharma Belt. "I would leave in the morning at eight o'clock. I would let her in, tell her how to lock up, and she would spend all day getting the protocols ready." The protocols written by David, Tony, Samir, and Denis needed to be prepared for distribution. Attention to detail was very important, particularly given the novelty of intravitreal injection. When Evelyn came home in the evening from a day at Roche, Lillian would be leaving, ready with the protocols to ship back to David in New York.

When you think of startup companies, the classic image that comes to mind is usually guys punching code in garages in Silicon Valley. With Eyetech, two ladies got the wheels turning typing up protocols in a guest bedroom in New Jersey.

MOVEMENT AFOOT

Strangely, Evelyn began finding the work she was doing for David more interesting than her day-to-day duties at her job. The idea of leaving began to gnaw at her. Getting out from under the bureaucracy was appealing. She could build her own team instead of just inheriting whoever was available. But there was one big sticking point: Included with her promotion was a major perk—her own parking space.

For ten years, Evelyn was forced to schlep over half a mile every morning from the general employees parking lot to the other side of the campus—rain, hail, sleet, or snow. This was not how she liked to enjoy the sensory bounty of the Garden State. It did nothing to enhance her mood at the start of the workday and only lengthened its end. But now, finally, she could roll almost right to the front door, to a place reserved for her use only. Her name was on it, a symbolic gesture that said, "You've arrived, Madam Director!" One that everyone at the company acknowledged. Joining Eyetech was one thing, but could she make this sacrifice?

To resolve this conundrum, Evelyn needed some elder counseling, so she sought her mother's advice. As luck would have it, or perhaps due to the workings of a higher power, her mother had recently seen a documentary on TV about successful people. What did they have in common? They took risks. Evelyn decided she was a risk-taker too. And as her mother pointed out, she could always go back to Big Pharma if Eyetech didn't pan out.

Just like a shrewd investor, Evelyn wanted to share the start-up risk, right up front. There was another person she wanted to bring with her to Eyetech, Kristine Curtiss, with an eye to appointing her clinical operations director. The two of them would be attending an upcoming oncology conference, ASCO, in New Orleans, and the trip back was the ideal place to pull Kristine aside to talk about the opportunity at Eyetech without someone from her employer overhearing. However, when the conference concluded, Kristine was adamant that a colleague join them for the taxi ride back to the airport. After Kristine made several attempts to get their associate, Evelyn finally got the courage to preempt the conversation, telling Kristine, "Look, we're not waiting. Just come with me. There's something I need to talk to you about." Remarkably, this terse ultimatum was the ideal introduction to her pitch.

In the cab, Evelyn laid out how she'd been moonlighting with Denis at Eyetech. Now, the time had come to accept a full-time position at the start-up. But it was a lot to take on. There was a need for another person; would she be interested? Evelyn thought Kristine was a long shot, at best. She expected this conversation to be just the start of an ongoing seduction, much like her own. To Evelyn's surprise, Kristine didn't hesitate, quickly responding, "I'm in."

Kristine's rationale captured the moment. As Evelyn recalls, Kristine elaborated, "The last time I didn't go with you and Denis, we were in Mexico, and there was a potential hurricane. And I didn't go with you and take the flight home. Instead, I took a bus for like ten hours through the back roads of Mexico with the rest of the gang." Evelyn was aghast. Kristine continued, "And it took me two days to get home! Meanwhile, you and Denis were home in like three hours."

It was clear, Kristine knew where the smart money was headed. Evelyn said she'd let Denis know that Kristine was in. A sense of relief passed through Evelyn: "We have the trifecta. We can do this." The only issue? Denis was stuck at the starting gate.

Casting his mind back to that period, Denis didn't share Evelyn's enthusiasm for joining a start-up. "I wasn't inspired at all," he recalls. On the cusp of turning fifty, he felt he was too old. If he envisioned a different future, it was retirement that came into focus. Not endless hours working toward an uncertain outcome. While Evelyn mused over the opportunity to put together her own team, Denis felt that was all he needed to do: assemble them and send them on their way. As for David's dream, he'd already "said no umpteen thousand times."

The team he'd put together was solid. In addition to Evelyn and Kristine, it included Loni da Silva. Loni brought expertise in the regulatory side of drug development. In her twelve years in pharma, Loni had worked her way up to a regulatory global leader. Her experience spanned an array of treatments, from antivirals and anti-infectives to oncology. She had been deeply involved with every indication relating to interferon, including the failed ophthalmological trial. When the aptamer from Gilead needed to go through approval processes around the world, Loni would know how to shepherd its every step. But before anything could happen, the team needed to jump ship. To this end, they assembled at Denis's house on a weekend to convince him to lead the way down the gangplank.

"It was a circular argument," explains Denis. "None of them would go because, they said, 'We'll only go if you go.' And I said, 'Well, no. You don't need me.'" Overhearing the increasingly heated conversation, Denis's wife came to the rescue. It was all new to her, as Denis hadn't discussed his situation—if he wasn't planning on leaving, what was there to talk about?

Denis's wife pointedly asked her husband, "What's stopping you going?" Having lived through so much with Denis, she felt like this was either a compelling sequel or a great final act. "You didn't want the ophthalmology program in Strasbourg, and you gave in to it. And years later, it's all coming together with a new company in ophthalmology." She summed it up: "This is clearly meant to be."

The collective wisdom of four women finally tipped the scales. Denis was on his way, too. Perhaps this was why earlier, he encountered his boss in that restaurant bathroom. It was a sign for him to let it all go.

Evelyn cruised into her dedicated parking spot the following Monday morning. It was a special day: her tenth anniversary at the big pharma company. And the day she was going to quit. When she approached the vice president to announce her decision, she was startled to learn that she was the third person to do so—Kristine and Denis had already beaten her to the punchline. After reassuring Evelyn that she could return to the company if this new eye drug venture ran aground, the vice president questioned Evelyn's true motivation, commenting, "The parking space wasn't close enough?"

Twenty years later, at her dentist's office, Evelyn recalls running into a former coworker from Roche. The exodus to Eyetech was still sorely remembered at the company. All three of them resigning that same day was "legendary" according to the woman. Even before Evelyn began her first full-time day at Eyetech, she was already receiving calls from others asking, "Can I join you?"

666—THE DEVIL MAY CARE (ACTUALLY)

The impetus behind the trio leaving Roche was David having signed a lease for the company's headquarters. Eyetech was no longer homeless. With about a dozen small offices along a corridor and a section of cubicles, the new office was modest in scale. Its location, however, was nothing short of grand. Unlike most start-up founders who established their companies in "Silicon Alley," as the area around the Flatiron Building on 5th Avenue and 23rd Street became known during the dot-com era, David had set his sights on midtown Manhattan and a building with a distinct pedigree. Everyone in New York knew 666 Fifth Avenue.

Three neon sixes emblazoned the building's corners on Fifty-Second and Fifty-Third Street at its crest of forty-one stories, glowing like devilish lapels on the shoulders of an impeccably shiny aluminum facade. Walking along New York's main thoroughfare, you could sense the numbers peering over the tops of other buildings, down to St. Patrick's Cathedral, reinforcing the sense that the city was the center of the universe, where God and his archrival perpetually faced off high above its hustling denizens.

For many of David's peers and particularly the elder statesmen of ophthalmology, Eyetech's address was distinctly symbolic. Being in cahoots with the pharmaceutical industry—especially for academics—was tantamount to working with the devil. It was almost as if by moving into the gleaming high-rise with its nefarious connotation, David was simultaneously acknowledging his shift to the dark side and thumbing his nose at the establishment. From David's point of view, working with the industry was the only way to make real progress. Big drug trials require big money. Ultimately, he would be vindicated, but in the meantime, his means of coping with acrimony from his fellow eye doctors was to keep his head down and focus on the work in front of him, despite being thirty-five floors in the sky.

Just four floors up from Eyetech, occupying the building's penthouse, was the Grand Havana Room, a private cigar lounge with a captivating view of the city. It was the kind of place one would join following a successful

IPO and years of profits, not before. An investor visiting Eyetech, after passing through the lobby with its sculptural waterfall and ceiling by the famed Japanese-American artist Isamu Noguchi, might be forgiven for thinking the fledgling company wasn't carefully preserving its working capital. However, once he or she entered the workspace on the thirty-fifth floor, that notion would be quickly abandoned in the flurry of activity.

Except possibly on the first day of occupancy.

Eyetech was never destined to be one of those start-ups that revolved around an endless game of air hockey that gets interrupted by hackathons and agile software scrums. While the company's leaders—David, Tony, and Samir—were deeply engaged in constructing trial protocols, dealing with the scores of doctors needed for the trials, and meeting with investors, the company's core personnel—pharmaceutical and health industry veterans, not straight-out-of-college coders—were tasked with setting up the office. Nonetheless, as former employees of a vast global enterprise with an abundance of support staff, the do-it-yourself mentality of a start-up was a shock.

"I remember the first day I had to push three or four boxes of my stuff up the freight elevator on a dolly," recalls Evelyn, "and I said to myself, 'What have you gotten yourself into?'" When she settled into her office, she got another surprise: David's executive assistant walked in, placed two pencils on her desk, and said, "Here's your office supplies."

For Denis, the disconnect between his former job and his new one was even greater. "I had always led teams," he notes, "but I didn't know the minutia of clinical operations and what's needed." Evelyn and Kristine, who were immediately engaged in setting up the first clinical studies, knew exactly how to put their boss to work. While the two women established standard operating procedures (SOPs) for the various components of the trials, they sent him, a senior VP, on errands to Staples. They needed folders, pens, and flex cards. When the pair asked him to get bankers boxes for files, he was stumped: "What have bankers got to do with this?"

Providentially, Kristine and Evelyn had worked their way up the ladder at Roche from clinical research associates to senior clinical research associates, then managers up to directors. With ten years behind them, they knew what to do from the bottom to the top and hit the ground running. Some days it was associate-level work; others they acted like managers; and sometimes, the work called for their director-level expertise. Their superpower was flexibility. However, they quickly reached the point where they were stretched too thin.

* * *

More employees were necessary to conduct the trials. While the initial team was busy creating the office around them, they were also hiring people to monitor the studies—those responsible for going to hospitals and other sites, ensuring all the standard processes were followed correctly. Over the next few weeks, Denis was aware of the offices and desks around him filling up with newly onboarded staff. But he was taken aback when Eyetech received a legal notice from his former employer, forbidding future hires to the new company. "I've brought four people," he remembers thinking. "How can they be sending me a cease and desist?"

It abruptly dawned on Denis that quite a few of the new people at the desks around him were also from his past company. Evelyn, Kristine, and Loni had continued to mine their networks for talent. Between them, they had almost a cumulative half a century in Big Pharma, so it's easy to understand why it was the first port of call for recruitment. When the trials eventually were underway, Eyetech was staffed with a number of former workers from their past company.

While Eyetech immediately complied with the cease and desist request, unfortunately for Denis, the pharma giant's behavior had consequences beyond the legal letter. He was applying for US citizenship, a process requiring documentation of all travel in and out of the country during his residency. Given the international nature of his role, he'd been relying on the company to assist him with information about all his globetrotting. Up to this point, they had been very cooperative. "Suddenly it was no. I was persona non grata," he remembers. He remembers he even received a call telling him he wasn't allowed on their premises, although the apologetic voice on the other end couldn't tell him why.

Despite the personal affront, when Denis discussed the letter with Harsha Murthy, now Eyetech's vice president, administration, Harsha, the lawyer, wasn't perturbed. He didn't think it amounted to much. His past company didn't do ophthalmology to any significant degree, so they weren't in competition. And besides, Eyetech had gotten the expertise it needed. Once again, being small and nimble paid off.

PUT TO THE TEST

After six years at GE Capital, Harsha was ready for something different. He'd enjoyed learning the ropes of how business gets done globally. It was highly instructive after being enmeshed in oversight at the SEC, as a kind of chief of staff to the chairman in Washington. But GE under Jack Welch was run in almost military fashion. When Harsha asked about advancing his career, he was informed he had the ability to one day run a multi-billion-dollar division, but he'd have to wait until his commanding officer was "killed in action or retired." By the end of the twentieth century, and a roll of financial skirmishes, the wait had been long enough.

As soon as he announced his availability, Harsha started receiving offers from start-ups. Then one day he received a call from Marty, who'd been tipped off about his employment status by a mutual acquaintance in finance. The idea of working for this new eye care company was appealing, especially as it was based in New York. Harsha had grown up in Columbus, Ohio, the son of an Indian physician. He studied political science and economics at Duke and then law at Stanford before feeling the pull of the city that never sleeps in the 1980s. At the turn of the millennium, he still felt it, even though the position at Eyetech would only pay a third of his GE income. However, there were stock options and the opportunity to test his skills across a wide spectrum of roles, unlike at GE where everyone had clearly defined duties according to rank.

First off, after the meeting with Gilead, Harsha did all the basic legal block and tackling, the certificate of incorporation, and bylaws. Once that was sorted out and Eyetech was up and running, he came on board officially, right after the trio from Roche. With the immediate need for a Phase 1 trial and the recruiting of personnel to conduct it, he quickly found himself in an HR position. The complexities of hiring world-class professionals in a very advanced field became apparent.

Over the course of the next year, he found himself entangled in all manner of delicate negotiations. "A lot of these guys were difficult to deal with," Harsha remembers learning as he became acquainted with the upper echelons of the pharma industry. "Some of these people wanted more money than David to come join the company." But giant egos made decision-making easier for Harsha: "That's just a nonstarter." He told them, "We can't have somebody who's here as a clinical consultant being paid more than the CEO." Several hires were considerably more nuanced. There were many elements to the job that were fungible, location being one. For one senior position, Harsha had to help sell the executive's house in California and get a mortgage for his new digs in New York.

Among the many hats he wore in the early days of the start-up, Harsha also found himself recruiting patients for the Phase 1B trial, which entailed just three injections at monthly intervals. In the end, this turned out to be the most rewarding experience. One patient suffering from AMD was a chef at a high-end restaurant. "He had been relegated to literally stirring the soup only," Harsha recounts, "because the restaurant said, 'We can't take the chance that you'll cut something in the wrong way, cut the vegetables the wrong way, or cut off your finger.'" Once the trial began, his sight improved remarkably. "By being on your therapy," the chef told Harsha, "I restored my sight to at least being legally sighted, and that allowed me to resume my duties." Another patient recruited by Harsha was a software engineer. Before the trial, she'd bought the biggest screen possible and blew up code to a huge font size and still couldn't read it. After a few shots, she, too, was back to work. To Harsha, the journeys of these patients were also morale boosters for the employees at Eyetech. It wasn't just another start-up peddling vaporware. People's lives were changed. Eyetech was creating hope. Who wouldn't want to get on board?

The first phase of trials was to test the safety of the drug, which at this point was known as Pegaptanib, a name derived from its chemical structure and mode of action: *peg* for polyethylene glycol, which improves stability and solubility; *apta* referring to the aptamer; and *nib* indicating it is an inhibitor of VEGF. It's not possible to embark on large-scale trials if the drug isn't found to be safe. So these initial trials were with very small numbers of patients. The trials also monitored the drug's effectiveness but not in an advanced way with randomized control groups. Still, the results were very encouraging.

In the first trial, there were five groups of three patients, and each group received a single dose of a different size. After three months, 80 percent of the patients showed stabilized or improved vision, and 27 percent could read more lines on an eye chart. For the next trial, ten patients received an intravitreal injection in the affected eye once a month for three months. Eight patients were tested at the end of the period, and approximately 88 percent had no further loss of vision and some improvement with 25 percent showing the ability to read fifteen or more additional letters on the Early Treatment Diabetic Retinopathy Study (ETDRS) eye chart.

Similarly, in the last trial, eleven patients received an injection in their affected eye once a month for three months. This time, the patients were also undergoing PDT in conjunction with the drug, getting the laser therapy just prior to the injection. In this case, 90 percent showed stabilization or improvement, and 60 percent were able to read fifteen more letters on the ETDRS eye chart, equivalent to three lines on the more familiar Snellen chart.

By the middle of 2001, it was clear that the drug had no apparent adverse effects as yet and showed tremendous promise as a treatment. The experiences of the patients Harsha had brought to the trial were the rule, not exceptions.

Throughout the trials, the office at 666 Fifth Avenue was filled up not only with the results—which in those days required physical storage on paper, meaning ever-expanding files crammed into filing cabinets—but also with the people running the operations. David's office, once the domain of just the CEO, now housed four others, squeezed in among his decorative antiques, which he installed in the very early days when appearances commanded more value than space. The fixtures were from India, imported by one of Samir's nonmedical entrepreneurial efforts, a furniture company complete with a warehouse in Chicago.

THE ULTIMATE THREAT—ALMOST

Simultaneously, as the company assembled its workforce and ran its first trials, it was also expanding its ranks of consultants. The culmination of this sixteen-month effort, which began shortly after the onset of the millennium—and included attracting very senior ex-executives from Merck and other pharma luminaries—was the first managerial retreat at 666 Fifth Ave on September 11, 2001.

The first sign of trouble appeared on the IBM PC of Lillian Vasquez. She was tuned into the online version of the *Today* show, such as it was in the pre-streaming era. "Oh, Harsha, a plane has crashed at the World Trade Center." Harsha paid little attention, thinking it was an accident, probably some small plane whose pilot had navigation trouble. Not exactly a common occurrence, but certainly not the first time this had happened in New York.

Despite the unfolding drama, Eyetech's COO was determined to remain focused on the matters at hand. In the company's small conference room, the assembled group remained diligently discussing the financial needs of the upcoming trial. But David couldn't help but feel a creeping sense of ill ease. "He just kept going through the material," remembers David about his earnest colleague, "and you could look at everyone's face, and everybody was shocked."

On a short break, David felt compelled to watch the events unfold on his computer with Peter Ernster, a former senior VP from Merck. They saw the second plane strike the South Tower of the World Trade Center. It was a chilling, unforgettable moment. "He said something I always remember," David recalls. "He said, 'The world has changed forever.'"

Also, during the break, Harsha checked in with Lillian. And when she said, "Another plane has hit," Harsha's blasé attitude, typical of New Yorkers, shattered.

Harsha immediately ran down the corridor to the corner office. Its view gave him a direct line of sight downtown to the tip of Manhattan. "I saw the smoke coming off the World Trade Center," he remembers. Alarmed, he relayed the news: "I went in and told everyone, this has happened, and we're being advised to evacuate because if this was an aerial attack, we'd be an easy target."

Harsha continues, "I brought everybody downstairs." He called the manager of the Omni Berkshire Place Hotel near the corner of Madison Avenue and Fifty-Second Street, with whom he had a relationship; it was the place where guests on *Saturday Night Live* stayed. Harsha explained the group had to evacuate and got them a conference room and lunch. It was the best way to calm nerves.

Cell phone systems, still relatively new, weren't handling the traffic. People couldn't communicate with their families. But the frazzled group discovered they had a work-around. Don Hodgkin, a consultant who brought his drug manufacturing expertise to the meeting, also came equipped with one of the original analog mobile phones, a giant archaic slab of electronics fondly known as a "brick." Made famous in the movie *Wall Street* by Gordon Gekko, it was a device that screamed machismo rather than practicality. But on this turbulent day, its antiquated tech proved superior, allowing the group to call the landlines in their homes—still prevalent at the time—one by one.

Around four o'clock, it seemed like nothing further was going to happen that day; but getting out of the city was troublesome. One of the first things the city did, just nine minutes after the second plane hit, was close all the bridges and tunnels connecting Manhattan. The subway was also shut down for a while along with intercity buses and Amtrak. And for the first time, the entire airspace over the US and Canada was emptied of planes.

One person who had a keen sense of the scale of the disaster was Katherine Burke, David's ophthalmic technician at Yannuzzi's practice who followed him to Eyetech. As soon as the second plane struck, she decided to evacuate immediately, picking up her pocketbook and clearing out. Her astute timing meant she was ahead of the crowds, taking advantage of public transportation before it was disrupted. She rode a bus to Ninety-Third Street and stocked up provisions at her local Key Food so she could hunker down for the duration.

A large portion of Eyetech's staff were based in New Jersey, having formerly been employed by Roche. The scene when they got to the Hudson River was chaotic. "It was very surreal," Evelyn remembers. "You saw people covered in dust. Their shoes, their suits. You knew they had been in the area where the towers went down. They had a shell-shocked look on their faces. We were all shocked, but you could see it was a different level of shock with them." An impromptu flotilla of boats—from small craft to the giant Circle Line tourist vessels—gathered to transport the swarm of people off the island.

Denis wasn't so lucky; he didn't make it back to New Jersey. Instead, he camped out at Katherine's place. Her stop at Key Food proved fortuitous. "I bought a lot of food," she says of her intuitive decision. "I thought a lot of people were going to come to my house. The only one who showed up was Denis." But after walking the whole way from Midtown, he stayed for two days, remaining in his suit without a change of clothes. As the nation tried to make sense of the catastrophe, Denis did his best to relieve Katherine of her overstocked pantry and fridge.

The out-of-town guests faced a similar predicament with civilian air traffic grounded for forty-eight hours, then flights resuming slowly with heightened airport security. Finding hotel accommodation was tricky. Peter Ernster, who had gone to college in New York, walked over to the

University Club and stayed there. Others, like Stuart Builder, managed to bunk with friends.

David walked back to his place on the Upper East Side through the eerily quiet streets, devoid of traffic and reclaimed by pedestrians. He and Maria went out to dinner at a local Indian restaurant. Their waiter had just done the reverse of David's commute on foot, walking over an hour and a half from an outer borough to get from his home to his job, facing the same effort again at his shift's end.

Eventually, the dust cleared, transportation resumed, and the sense of immediate crisis began to fade, but September 11 shook up the company in some unexpected ways. A consensus formed that it was time to move from 666 Fifth Avenue—it was too crowded, and the company had outgrown it. Also, for the New Jersey staffers, the struggle to get back home on that tragic day left a lingering feeling that it would be better to be closer to New Jersey transit.

While the entire country was left processing what the attack meant and how to respond, a new threat emerged for David and his company. Ironically, this new peril was a direct result of their success. Once Eyetech made the success of its initial trials public, the sleeping giant stirred. Apparently, it finally dawned on Genentech that there really was potential to develop its anti-VEGF molecule for ophthalmic use.

It was time to put the pedal to the metal!

Chapter 6

THE BIGGEST BIOTECH FIRM IN THE GARMENT DISTRICT

Genentech entering the race had a surprisingly positive effect on Eyetech. It wasn't a sharpening of focus or an amping up of determination since the small company was already moving at breakneck speed. It may seem contrary to common sense, but having a big, established competitor helped Eyetech raise more money. And lots of it. Quickly. In the nick of time, too. Running the next phases of drug trials was going to be vastly more complicated, involving many more patients—about a thousand of them—and a hundred-plus locations around the globe, adding up to an enormous expense. The best guess? About $42 million. Together with other operating costs, the fledging outfit would likely burn through at least $65 million by the end of 2002. To be safe, the next round of fundraising, Series C, needed to reach $75 million. This would be a significant undertaking even for experienced businessmen. Appealing to investors at this level was a whole new challenge for the three eye doctors.

Call it beginner's luck, but one of the key investors David, Tony, and Samir solicited was a newbie in the world of pharmaceutical investing. "It was the craziest thing," recounts Srini Akkaraju. "Literally the first company I met with on the very first day of my job as an investor was

Eyetech." The second craziest thing about the newly minted JP Morgan banker: Srini's previous job was at Genentech.

Fresh from the West Coast, Srini had gained an MD-PhD at Stanford and then dabbled in the start-up world as a researcher, where he got reverse recruited. In trying to lure a Genentech employee into his new business venture, Srini instead was led into the arms of the biotech giant. "When the start-up didn't go forward," Srini explains, "that guy pulled me into Genentech." Having decided to follow the money, Srini devoted his brain power not to the laboratory but to the business development side of biotech. Eventually, this stirred a desire to get into investing. And that drew him to JP Morgan Partners in New York, just a short walk from Eyetech's energized office.

At first, when he heard the name, Srini thought Eyetech was a medical device company, like most of the firms in the ophthalmological space. But when his new boss, Damion Wicker, invited him to a meeting with David, he quickly discovered Eyetech was in therapeutics, like Genentech. But unlike his previous employer, Eyetech moved at New York speed. This was immediately evident in how rapidly its founder spoke. "David talks like a hundred miles an hour," Srini explains. "The guy speaks while breathing in and out. Because he doesn't give you the gap to force in a question, you have to get a crowbar to ask him something."

Not wishing to be bamboozled by fast-talking East Coasters, Srini quickly set about doing his due diligence. There was good evidence to back up David's claims. "Eyetech presented me their Phase 1 data, which showed you get drying up," Srini said about the leaky vessels in wet AMD being affected by the drug. "They showed it had some effect, at least stasis on visual acuity, maybe a little benefit."

It was familiar territory. At Genentech, even though his focus was licensing deals, Srini was also the project leader for a cancer antibody and knew the company's anti-VEGF work, including its potential wet AMD application. Although still focused on oncology, Genentech had had a change of heart about ophthalmology. At some point in the four years following David's failed quest to work with them, the company apparently did an about-face and seemed to have concluded that injecting people in their eyeballs wasn't so outrageous after all, and maybe there was a market. In fact, rather than considering a second eye simply a spare part, they evidently started considering the fact that everyone has two eyes possibly meant the unrealized market size was actually double. And perhaps they should go ahead and develop an ophthalmic drug on their own rather than with a partner.

What the beginner banker didn't immediately recognize, despite being in touch with the medical research landscape, was that David was playing the investment field. "There was a lot of interest," David recalls about the beginning of Series C. "We had multiple term sheets (the non-binding framework outlining an agreement)—four or five—and maybe twenty syndicate members interested. JP Morgan was one of the finalists." Damion Wicker, however, didn't share his new junior associate's naivete. At the concluding meeting of their investment courtship, David recalls that the bankers were very nervous about the competition; they thought they might lose the deal: "The two things I remember was getting called to the JP Morgan office at night where Damion said, 'Everybody puts their cell phones down. And you can't call in the bathroom to the other place and try to negotiate. We leave here with a deal.'" The ultimatum worked. "We did that," affirms David, "but after we delayed faxing it over, then the next day he sent Srini over to our office with the actual paper to sign."

SEEING DOUBLE (IT TAKES TWO TO VERIFY)

As leaders of the Series C financing, JP Morgan's key goal was to entice other investors to follow suit. The April 2001 ARVO meeting in Fort Lauderdale, Florida, which Srini attended with Eyetech, presented him the opportunity to ask key opinion leaders about the biology and pathophysiology of wet AMD. To prominent research specialists, he queried, "Why do you think anti-VEGF makes sense? What else do we know about what's driving this disease process? How long is this disease going to last? And what do you think about the Eyetech data?" The expert insights were illuminating.

Then the spotlight shone in another direction. Genentech presented some preclinical data on what was then known as ranibizumab, its monoclonal antibody fragment. Srini took note. Here was a different kind of anti-VEGF, and the results were similar to Eyetech's. "For me," Srini remembers, "it was critically important, validating data." It wasn't so much that Srini doubted Eyetech's claims, but "Genentech also showed the same kind of effect in the same patient population with the same mechanism." In other words, Eyetech's effort wasn't a fluke. Great science is repeatable.

Not surprisingly, as the holder of a PhD, Srini's aim was to produce an investment thesis. A fully fleshed-out rationale for investors to understand the value and risk inherent in Eyetech. Only one element still clouded his ability to reach a conclusion. What was the true size of the opportunity?

It was the same old problem. Looking back into past ophthalmological therapeutics was no help in projecting future outcomes. Focused on the back of the eye, Eyetech with AMD was different. And glancing sideways at the newly developed competition was no help either. Around the same time Eyetech licensed the aptamer, the Canadian company QLT brought Visudyne to market.

Essentially, Visudyne was a halfway point between laser and therapeutics. Administered intravenously by a catheter in the arm, about ten minutes later the Visudyne collects inside the abnormal vessels in the eye. After a contact lens is placed in the eye, the Visudyne reacts when a laser strikes an abnormal vessel in the retina, causing the Visudyne there to transform into a substance that closes off the vessel without harming surrounding tissue. It represented the commercialization of photodynamic therapy (PDT). But what was troubling to an investment guy like Srini was why Visudyne didn't have more sales. In its first year, it garnered an estimated $200 million. Granted, Visudyne was just for a subset of AMD sufferers, but still, surely with a solution to a problem as big as AMD, there was more money to be made?

Just because there wasn't an easy answer didn't mean there was no answer. Especially as Genentech was now in the game. Why would the Bay Area juggernaut pursue an AMD treatment if it wasn't expecting to be handsomely rewarded? So Srini and JP Morgan Partners crunched their own numbers. "We did a bottom-up analysis," Srini recounts. "What's the actual incidence? What's the prevalence of wet AMD patients? How many of those would actually be treated if eligible and we had this kind of market share, this kind of market penetration?" His conclusion loudly echoed Marty's: "This is a billion-dollar-plus drug."

In DME, leaky blood vessels in the retina are caused by chronically high blood sugar levels. David and Tony's plan was to conduct a separate set of DME trials about six months behind the AMD work, with a launch into the market, also half a year later. This added to the necessary financial outlay but also sweetened the outcome, increasing the potential market by around two hundred thousand new patients annually in the US, and possibly two to three million globally.

To justify raising $75 million, Srini focused on three key attributes: "One, David is a retinal specialist, and he had great people around him; his team was fantastic. Two, the fact that Genentech had the same data in a small patient population. And number three, our bottoms-up analysis said that this was actually a much more interesting market opportunity than people were giving credit." In addition, he saw a unique commercial advantage, heightened by his experience at ARVO. Retinal specialists were a small and readily accessible group. That meant you could effectively market the drug with just a modest and manageable sales force—something a start-up like Eyetech could easily build. With just thirty-five to forty people, Srini felt "you can go get every single retinal specialist out there."

Indeed, in this regard, Eyetech had a considerable advantage over its larger, deep-pocketed rival—Eyetech was run by ophthalmologists and led by a retinal specialist. Genentech had no such concentration of expertise on hand. Not only could Eyetech easily connect to the drug's audience, but they could communicate with a level of understanding impossible for the biotech giant. Ironically, this advantage also contained an element of risk. Doctors aren't renowned for their business acumen. Internally, JP Morgan was nervous about David's unproven ability as a first-time CEO. He might be fine for getting the drug through the trials, but could he handle the non-medical challenges he would certainly face running a company? Could he execute an exit strategy when the time came for investors to recoup?

Besides the data, the ARVO meeting made one thing very clear: The race against Genentech was now public—especially to the audience that mattered most. What was Eyetech's key advantage? Oddly enough, size. Being small made the company more nimble than its lumbering competitor. But would speed be more important than strength? Genentech was awash in money and resources, and Eyetech had yet to raise the capital for the coming crucial rounds of trials. However, for its size, the fledgling firm punched way above its weight class. The personnel who had run the interferon trial for Roche, Genentech's majority shareholder, were now with Eyetech. Although brand new, Eyetech alone had the institutional knowledge of how to run a global ophthalmological trial. There was no learning curve and no bureaucratic friction. Already out in front, Eyetech only needed the financial fuel to power it forward to become the winner. This was a compelling story to tell potential backers.

Srini wasn't the only investor conducting due diligence. Eyetech's first venture supporters, SV Life Sciences, had expanded to include an experienced scientist in addition to its financial team. Mike Ross garnered multiple academic credentials starting with a bachelor's degree in chemistry at Dartmouth College, then a PhD in biochemistry at the California Institute of Technology (Caltech), and a postdoctoral fellowship at Harvard before becoming Genentech's tenth employee in 1978. After eleven years, Mike left the pioneering biotech firm to become CEO at a string of start-ups, bringing his well-rounded expertise to SV just in time to investigate how Eyetech's approach would stand up against his former employer's new drug. After talking with Tony, Mike concurred with Srini. Although both drugs involved the same mechanism, Eyetech's pegaptanib offered a more precise attack which should, in theory, be more efficient and pose fewer safety risks. All things considered; it remained a solid investment.

INJECTING AN ELEMENT OF RISK

One area of uncertainty remained. And uncertainty to investors means risk. It's a financial truism that there is no reward without risk, and generally greater risk means greater reward. A new drug in a new market is already plenty risky. What Srini wanted to do was eliminate any unnecessary unpredictability.

Injecting medication once or three times into twenty people's eyes is one thing. Clearly Eyetech had no problem facilitating small trials. But doing that to one thousand-plus people around the world every six weeks for just over a year is many orders of magnitude more difficult. Once David's team had lined up the doctors participating in the trial, could Eyetech actually make a steady supply of its drug at scale?

Pegaptanib sodium, which Eyetech code-named EYE-001, an aptamer, was still a therapeutic novelty at the turn of the millennium. No FDA-approved aptamer was yet in existence. This folded-up nucleic acid requires highly specialized manufacturing processes—an origami-like convergence of intricate bioprocess encompassing a number of molecular biology techniques, chemical synthesis, purification, and analytical characterization to assess its stability. "Aptamers are this whole other sort of class of drugs," Srini succinctly explains, thinking back to the manufacturing reality of over two decades ago, "that turned out to be a pain in the ass to make."

Nobody at Eyetech could tell him how they were going to produce the very essence of the company—the drug—at scale. While Srini had abundant confidence in David and his team's ability to conduct the trials, how they were going to fill all the syringes in the hands of ophthalmologists around the planet remained a mystery. When they did the interferon trial for Roche, the Swiss conglomerate had been manufacturing drugs for a century. Eyetech? It had only been on the scene for a New York minute.

Again, Srini's connection to Genentech alumni proved invaluable. "So I called up my buddy Robert Baffi, who was the guy in manufacturing at Genentech." As fortune would have it, Baffi had departed Genentech a few months ahead of Srini to become the chief technology officer at BioMarin, a company with no interest in ophthalmology nor currently developing any aptamers. When Srini asked Baffi for a favor, Baffi was able to assist without any conflicts of interest. With BioMarin's permission, he took time off and visited a manufacturing facility in Colorado, near Denver, and returned with some good news and some bad news.

The bad news: Making the aptamer was very expensive. Not a surprise given the complexity and lack of precedent. The good news: Because injecting directly in the eye meant using highly concentrated solutions, in doses of just a few milliliters, a single manufacturing run could produce all the material necessary for the global trial. Phew!

While the novice investor was enthusiastic about Eyetech, Srini was keenly aware of the dark shadow hovering over the financial arena. By the end of 2000, the dot-com bust had seen most publicly traded internet companies lose about 75 percent of their stock price from their peaks in March. CNN Money dubbed those downhill nine months the "$1.755 trillion dot-com investing lesson." Speculators were licking their wounds, not reaching into their pockets. Ultimately, the bear market continued until 2002, and the NASDAQ wouldn't hit 5000 again for another fifteen years. In 2001, unlike the beginning of the previous year, when it came to raising $75 million, having the word *tech* in the name of the company wasn't exactly an asset.

But Srini's due diligence (and perhaps his beginner's luck) paid off. It also may have been that Eyetech's blindness treatment was a rare shining star in a dim night sky for investors—particularly when its full potential dawned on financiers at the receiving end of one of David's exuberant pitches, delivered with both professorial finesse and the conviction of a man giving sight to the blind. After a veritable meteor shower of positive data on slides flying by at rotoscopic speed to keep pace with David's verbal fusillade, what moneyman could possibly maintain a flicker of hesitation? Despite the economic environment, raising the $75 million happened in the blink of an eye. In a few short months, after contributing $35 million, JP Morgan Partners was joined by Merrill Lynch, MPM Capital, BB Biotech Ventures, Alta Partners, and Eyetech's original investor, the SV Life Sciences Fund, to raise what one pundit called "an eye-popping" $108.5 million in Series C. This meant having an extra $33.5 million—just in case—and was enough to garner the attention of *The Wall Street Journal* on August 7, 2001. At the time, this was the third-largest round of venture capital financing ever obtained by a biopharmaceutical firm. "All this demand came out of the woodwork," Srini remembers. "There ended up being like $150 million of demand; we weren't able to put it all in the term sheet."

The due diligence performed a dual service. Not only did Srini establish a sound investment thesis, but his investigation provided a crash course on running a $100 million business to the three doctors—David, Samir, and Tony. "It was clear to me," Srini reflects on the experience, "that they were learning about their drug and what they were going to do with it in the process of diligence." Indeed, Srini had spent so much time at Eyetech, that once the term sheet for the investment deal was signed and he was appointed to the company's board, David wondered if he could see less of him. As Srini remembers it, the Eyetech CEO told him, "We can't do our jobs with how much time you spend over here."

For the first-time investor, it was comforting to acknowledge that the Eyetech team, as students of business, felt they had absorbed enough wisdom to manage on their own. David turned out to be both a rapid-fire professor and a quick study.

A MUCH SOFTER SELL

The one part of David's life that didn't progress at breakneck speed was his relationship with Maria. The pair enjoyed travel, and Maria occasionally accompanied David on his trips to visit investigating doctors participating in the drug trials. Naturally, this gave David an opportunity to display his intimate knowledge of local restaurants around the world. Maria shared David's interest in good food, although with considerably less obsession. What they talked about over dinner was of more significance than the sensations crossing their taste buds. They grew closer, becoming more deeply involved in each other's lives, and developing a bond that lent a stillness to the center of their tumultuous careers.

Living together seemed like the natural next step in their relationship. Maria moved into David's apartment on New York's Upper East Side. In contrast to David's ongoing quest to stymie blood at the back of the eye, he had, in his heart, reached a conclusion: He had found his forever.

For a man accustomed to giving public presentations and lectures in auditoriums, he offered a simple, intimate proposal on the couple's couch: "Will you marry me?" The only moment of haste was the speed with which Maria answered, "Yes."

FAST MONEY! FAST TRACK!

David suddenly found himself with a large pile of investors' money in hand. It was all systems go. Importantly, the potential of Eyetech's drug wasn't only recognized by its backers. Given the name "Macugen" by Samir's wife, Arti, an anesthesiologist imbued with a large dose of creativity, it felt more substantial. This evaluation in status was reinforced when Macugen was awarded "fast track" status by the FDA. This designation is reserved for drugs the agency deems to be of high importance with the promise to address serious unmet medical needs. In practice, this means more frequent communication between the agency and the company plus eligibility for accelerated approval and priority review, which can significantly shorten the typically lengthy bureaucratic processes involved in New Drug Applications (NDAs).

Of all the decisions David made, day in and day out, the single most impactful one was without doubt compressing the Phase 2 and 3 trials into a single endeavor. Denis summed it up this way: "If David hadn't have done that. Macugen would've never got there first." This unorthodox approach also came with a high degree of risk.

Normally, the two trial phases serve distinct purposes. Phase 2 trials tend to be smaller—a few dozen to a few hundred patients—with the goal of determining the optimal dosage as a proof of concept and noting any side effects. The next phase goes wide—with many hundreds, often thousands of participants—seeking to understand the efficacy more broadly in statistically robust ways and in contrast to placebos or other drugs. Because of the increased scope, Phase 3 trials are of greater duration, usually several years, and they also monitor longer-term effects of drugs. These attributes make them a mandatory and very costly component of the drug approval process. But Phase 3 is absolutely critical for the drug to reach the market.

Although combining the two isn't unheard of, it is highly unusual. The kind of behavior that can put investors on edge. In Srini's words, it's "definitely a higher risk push on the accelerator kind of strategy." In the case of Macugen, this acceleration saved eighteen to twenty-four months. Vital for the drug to be the first to market.

For drug development to stay inside investors' comfort zones, it's best to reduce the risk level before going into the expensive Phase 3 trials, which means doing a robust Phase 2 trial. When that happens, the results are more predictive. According to the Biotechnology Innovation Organization (BIO), the industry's trade association, around 63 percent of drugs make it through Phase 1. It's the second phase where the shakeout happens, with only about 30 percent passing the test. In this scenario, the sequence is almost an hourglass shape, with a little better than 50 percent of the Phase 2 survivors producing positive results in Phase 3. Those that make it through the final test have about an 85 percent chance of being approved by the FDA. When you multiply all the risks together from beginning to end, a drug has slightly less than a one in ten chance of reaching the market.

But, as Srini reflects, in Eyetech's case, David's decision compounded the gamble: "Since we're going straight into it, we're combining all the risks." Still, he felt the data from Phase 1 and the corroboration by Genentech's data meant EYE-001 was strong enough to justify the velocity.

In hindsight, David feels the success probabilities are more of a crapshoot: "When you do a new mechanism of action in a novel compound, I don't think there are any layups."

Regardless of the odds, Eyetech's approach to the trials was totally run-and-gun. "It was the fastest recruitment in a retina trial ever," reminisces Tony. "That record has not yet been broken." This velocity, according to Tony, was partly due to "David driving it, and the other part was there was nothing out there. This was a really exciting, promising lead for patients and investigators."

Investigators in drug trials are usually physicians—in this case, retinal specialist ophthalmologists. They find and recruit participants and then ensure that the trial is conducted according to the study protocol at the site, or center, for which they are responsible, very often their own practice or clinic.

You might think for a trial spread across the globe, just getting the message out would be arduous. But as Srini had noted, the retinal world was small and one frequently traversed by David and Tony who were fixtures on its lecture circuit, spreading the anti-VEGF story, from the very compelling preclinical data to the early clinical results. "Every two or three weeks, we're at another meeting giving a talk," explains David. "And you meet people. Most of them much older. We were like the young guys on the tour. Cleveland, LA, Barcelona, wherever. We knew the top person in every city." So, as the new kid on the block, David would call these revered doctors, telling them, "We'd like you to be a center," and the old-timers were flattered; it was like being invited to a party with a much hipper crowd than their cronies.

GETTING ON "THE LIST"

In evaluating drugs, speed is a relative term. Inception to approval is an onerous process, averaging somewhere from eight to twelve years. With people's health and lives at stake, it's not hard to see why. By comparison, other products under the FDA's purview, such as processed foods, have greatly compressed timelines and can hit the market in a matter of months or just a few years. Plus Eyetech, looking at a global market, was set to conduct trials in North America alongside Europe, South America, Africa, the Middle East, and Australia, potentially adding more time and complexity. Throughout all these regions, maintaining consistency was paramount. At the end of the trial, the conclusions needed to be as generally applicable as possible.

This means the first step in the process needed to be rigorous. It all starts with ensuring you're studying the right population, which is a twofold undertaking. The first step is establishing the correct criteria for inclusion, and the next step is educating the practitioners manning the study's entry points—retinal specialists at 117 leading medical centers around the world—on how to recognize someone's is eligibility.

Wet AMD has three main subtypes, each with different kinds of lesions under the fovea; it was important to study them all. Additionally, the lesions vary considerably in size and possess different characteristics. All these diverse attributes were deemed worthy of inclusion. However, if a patient had previously received subfoveal laser therapy or suffered significant scarring or atrophy, they were ruled out.

Another key requirement for a patient to be deemed acceptable was their baseline of visual acuity, so the drug's effect can be measured over time. In the parlance of drug trials, the change in visual acuity is called "the primary endpoint," the single most important piece of the data puzzle. Again, the desire was to understand the outcome across a wide range of impairment. This meant anyone whose eyesight in their worse eye fell between 20/40 and 20/320 was acceptable—in other words, patients who need to stand at half the normal distance from an eye chart to read the letters to highly impaired AMD sufferers who must be so close to an eye chart they need to read it like it's a book and everyone in between. Their less affected eye had to be at least 20/80 or better, so newspaper headlines are readable but perhaps not the stories below. Of course, the eye chart in question had to conform to a standard, too. The ETDRS version was chosen because it was more accurate and also used in Visudyne's trials, and that would simplify the statistical analysis for easier comparison. Five letters on the ETDRS are equal to one line of visual acuity.

Before enrollment, the level of patients' impairment needed to be carefully recorded: not only how many lines on an eye chart could they read but also their subtype of AMD and the characteristics of any lesions they had. Eyetech engaged the Wilmer Eye Institute at Johns Hopkins University School of Medicine to review angiograms of each patient's affected eye to create a global, centralized standard for vetting patients and monitoring them. In the days before digital imaging technology gained traction in medicine, this meant FedEx was kept very busy, and became a hefty line item on the budget.

The task of training and certifying the clinicians and their staff who were examining patients at all the different sites fell into the lap of Katherine. "Usually, when you get your eyes checked at various places, the room is different, the light is different, the chart is different, the lenses, everything's different," elaborates Katherine. "I had to make sure they all did the vision testing and recording the same way, that all the equipment was standardized, and they were using the same lenses." Although the interferon trial provided a precedent, this new trial was on a far greater scale. "We had sites all over the world—South America, North America, all over Europe, South Africa, and Australia. I had to really invent this whole thing." Part of Katherine's creativity was putting together a team that could cover some of the territory: "I went to a lot of sites, but I couldn't do it all."

DON'T WORRY, IT WON'T HURT

In addition to the scale, there was an even greater challenge with this trial. The drug was to be injected intravitreally—directly into the vitreous humor, the clear gel-like substance between the lens and the retina. As mentioned previously, this wasn't unheard of in the world of ophthalmology, particularly with antivirals for CMV retinitis afflicting patients with weakened immune systems. But for most eye doctors, it was an uncommon procedure, at best, and still regarded as rather unorthodox. For many years, sticking needles in eyes was considered outright heresy. Ophthalmic textbooks warned of dire consequences when the vitreous was invaded, as it invariably led to the formation of scar tissue, which would then contract and dislodge the retina, pulling it off the back of the eye. Ironically, this was one reason why laser proved so popular: It permitted surgeons to operate inside the eye without having to first penetrate it.

As a resident at Johns Hopkins, David had been exposed to the use of intravitreal injections in very controlled laboratory settings. David's mentor, the esteemed Mort Goldberg, chairman of the university's prestigious Wilmer Ophthalmological Institute, had used intraocular drug delivery while at the Illinois Eye and Ear Infirmary in the late 1970s. Even Goldberg had reservations about this drug administration method before he gradually came around and began using it with antibacterials, antivirals, and corticosteroids for anti-inflammatory treatments. However, as none of these drugs were specifically developed for ophthalmological purposes, the technique had never been part of an FDA approval process. This caused two very practical problems for the Eyetech team: 1) devising an entirely new testing protocol and 2) familiarizing doctors with the injection procedure while preparing them to address patients' concerns. While no one wants to go blind, getting that first injection in your eye is intimidating.

Years later, reflecting on intravitreal treatments, Goldberg appreciates that David "had the brilliance to apply it to a totally new chemical approach, the anti-VEGF approach." At the time, however, David's stroke of inspiration became Katherine's headache. "Out of all those doctors," she recollects with a tinge of exasperation, "I would say probably 75 percent had never done it. They didn't even know what to do." But the Eyetech team quickly rose to the challenge. "We designed these kits—the speculum, the Betadine, how to prep the eyes—so they wouldn't get an infection." Well, that was the theory, in practice. Like so much in life, it was a little more complicated.

In fact, at one point Eyetech had struck a deal with the Draper Laboratory to work on the problem. Spun off from MIT, the Boston-based nonprofit specializes in designing advanced technological solutions for healthcare, energy, national security, and space exploration. Most famous for developing the Apollo Guidance Computer that safely sent astronauts to the moon and back, they wanted a shot at the orb closest to our brains. David can't forget the finale to their tantalizing pitch: "If we can put men on the moon, don't you think that we can deliver drugs to the back of the eye?" Ultimately, they failed. But fortunately, David had success with a more down-to-earth approach, by bringing familiar talent in-house.

Emmett Cunningham, a fellow ophthalmologist who had known David since their medical school days together at Johns Hopkins in the early 1980s, was brought on board at Eyetech as employee number twenty. "That's what was printed on my pay stub," he reflects with a trace of humor. As the company advanced toward the large Phase 3 trial, Emmett set to work with Denis to head up safety. When Emmett saw the infection rate of endophthalmitis in the early trial stages, it raised his eyebrows. "My recollection was that they had sixteen cases or a 1.6 percent rate of endophthalmitis, which would not have been acceptable. If one in fifty or one in a hundred patients got a severe blinding eye infection, this would not have moved forward." Despite the thorough protocol, clearly, something was going astray. It was up to Emmett to find out what it was and how to fix it. He had to dive deep: "We needed to understand, first of all, what's happening at each of these sites, each of these infections."

Emmett reached out to Chris Ta, an ophthalmologist specializing in microbiology who is now a professor at Stanford. "We paid Chris to go to every site every time there was an infection and to do a full protocol review," explains Emmett. "So this was very expensive—a business-class ticket all over the world, a few days in hotel, and then his hourly rate. It was probably twenty or thirty thousand dollars per case of endophthalmitis just to get to the bottom of it." Although costly, this extreme diligence uncovered a huge number of protocol violations. Chris discovered that doctors weren't sterilizing the surface of the eye properly and often failed to use a speculum. "If you're trying to inject an eye and the patient's blinking," he elaborates, "without a speculum, there are lots of bacteria on the lids that'll just get in the path of the needle and then get into the eye."

There was another more complex issue that emerged in Chris's investigations, one that revealed a more nuanced, ingrained mistrust of intravitreal injections. Ironically, doctors were taking an unnecessary precaution, an additional procedure known as prophylactic anterior chamber paracentesis. Because they were worried about adding extra liquid into the eyeball with each dose of Macugen and raising the pressure of the fluids in the eye, they preemptively extracted some fluid from the front of the eye. In reality, increased pressure wasn't much of an issue. So doctors were essentially doubling the risk of infection by poking two needles in the eye rather than just one.

"We had to teach the world how to do it," summarizes Emmett. At first, this meant Chris counseling the doctors at the sites with problems about what they did wrong. This grew into teleconferences with investigators to bring them up to speed and presentations at ophthalmic meetings. Ultimately, Emmett crafted the first guidelines on the correct approach to intravitreal injections to be published and circulated. The result of this effort was stunning. In the second year of the trial, the rates of infection plummeted, by a factor of ten. When the Eyetech team reported the good news, it sent shock waves throughout the ophthalmological community.

"I got a call," recounts Emmett, "from three very famous ophthalmologists, and they incorrectly accused me openly of hiding cases of endophthalmitis. They said, 'There's no way this rate could have dropped like that.'" The conversation turned unpleasant: "I kind of had a screaming match with them. I gave them the 'How dare you accuse me of this?'" No doubt everyone had patient safety at the forefront of their minds, but Emmett notes how this reaction was part of why they were successful: "That's how incredulous the field was that we could do this and scale it. At the end of the day, the reason that doctors accepted it was that there were just no other options."

That was only half the problem solved. As a double-masked (eye-related studies avoid using the term *blind*), controlled trial, a statistically significant group of patients had to receive a placebo. Swallowing a counterfeit pill that looks exactly like the real thing isn't hard to do. But injecting a person's eyeball? Unnecessarily introducing a fake drug into a patient's eye by needle, even using the specially devised kits, still carried some risk, which wasn't palatable to the Eyetech team and no doubt would be a hard sell to wary ophthalmologists. Instead, the control group had an empty syringe, without a needle attached, pressed against their eyeball. In short, they received a mock injection. This required teaching doctors a magician-like sleight of hand, preventing the patient from noticing the absence of the needle, then using enough pressure to be convincing but without hurting them. It no doubt helped that the recipients' sight was impaired in the first place.

To further reduce any bias, not only did the patient need to be ignorant of the dosage (or lack of dosage) administered, but so, too, did the investigational staff—all the doctors and medical workers measuring and recording the patients' response to the treatments. In the terminology of clinical trials, they were "masked." This meant the injections—whether sham or real—had to be given by an "unmasked" doctor who was not treating or monitoring the patient but could ensure the dosage was correct. With treatments occurring every six weeks, across four groups (the control group and groups receiving either 0.3 mg, 1 mg, or 3 mg per injection), the need to maintain secrecy was paramount. "Nobody knows who's getting what," Katherine explains. And the study coordinators were even more strict, according to her: "[They] were, my God, like the police. They wouldn't let you see anything. We saw clean data—you get printouts—but they're only numbers of people. There's no demographics. Not even male or female."

APPROACHING THE FINISH LINE

Not only were the trials cloaked in secrecy, but the data were also randomized and stratified. This helped balance out the representation of the different subtypes of AMD in addition to eliminating biases. Handling all the data was IDDI, a data management company, founded by Marc Buyse, with deep expertise in clinical trials. But even though everything was stored in a centralized database, inputting the information was a new experience for the staff at the study centers. On top of that, the now-standard ophthalmological imaging technology, optical coherence tomography, was still in its infancy, and the speedy and highly accurate generations that revolutionized the diagnosis of retinal disease only arrived in clinics in 2006. All of which added to the curriculum Katherine and her team had to teach to the clinical study centers around the world. Sometimes, this entailed going to individual practices, but often, it meant lecturing to large groups. "I did massive ones," Katherine recounts. "We did one in UCLA; there were like 150 people. We had all these optometrists I was working with. We'd bring examiners into each room, and they had to demonstrate they knew how to do it. It was kind of inventing the wheel." In venues outside the US, interpreters were added to the mix. "You'd have simultaneous translation, like at the UN."

Speed being as much of a concern to David as accuracy, he hired an in-office travel agent to streamline the grueling amount of travel needed to spread the clinical trial knowledge in those pre-Zoom days. The woman was Caribbean, and her uplifting demeanor reminded Katherine of the queen of TV psychics, Miss Cleo, a clairvoyant for the Psychic Readers Network. Her travel itineraries were often as much a matter of chance as a paranormal prediction, as she frequently misunderstood and confused destinations. "She would send people to the wrong place," explains Katherine. "Instead of going to Charlottesville, Virginia, she'd send you to Charlotte, North Carolina." Not only that, if she got a bad feeling about a certain flight—that it might crash—she would try to switch it. This mystical approach to transportation drove David nuts: "I'm like, you can't do that. I need to be there earlier. You can't make a flight six hours later because you think the plane's going to go down." It's one thing to randomize your trial data; it's another entirely to randomize your travel arrangements.

Despite the difficulties, the pace was unrelenting. "David was the force behind recruitment," asserts Tony. "There were a bunch of innovations that David came up with." The one that Eyetech team members felt had the greatest impact was also the simplest. "We had a tally board," Tony remembers. It was instrumental in motivating all the highly competitive, type-A doctors. In a newsletter that went out every few weeks, "they could see who was enrolling the most patients."

Updating the tally, prominently posted in David's office, acquired a ceremonial quality, as he insisted the responsibility lay solely with the trial manager. "David would only want Jill to put the number on the board," concedes Katherine. "She would put the number of patients on it every time one would get recruited. But no one else could do it. Only Jill." Not only was there a visual record of progress, but whenever there was an enrollment, a bell would be rung. It added to the sense of communal excitement, a reminder that they were moving full speed ahead. The tally was revised continuously, often hourly, whenever a patient anywhere around the world was randomized. "So, we'd have 53 patients, and as soon as there'd be another one, she'd go up there, erase it, put 54 patients." Katherine remembers it as the focal point of progress: "We were always looking at the board. Oh, we got 97! Oh my God! We have 180!"

David also added another sensory experience to the office—one that affected both taste buds and competitive drive. "I just filled the refrigerator with tons of Coca-Cola," David recalls with satisfaction. "All you can drink for free." With his own legendary consumption, he was clearly leading by example. However, the unbridled success of this initiative alarmed one of the board members: "We come to the board meeting, and one of the board members says, 'You can't give out free Coca-Cola. That's expensive!' And we have a fight at the board meeting, and Marty and I are like, 'Are you kidding me?'" In the years since Eyetech, providing all manner of creature comforts in the office has become de rigueur. "But it was so weird to me," David says of his experience. "Having to deal with this penny-pinching was ridiculous. You need to hire great people and treat them well."

The time came when the trial was almost fully enrolled. There was just one patient remaining. "The patient had an appointment on August 3," Katherine remembers. The problem? Evelyn was determined the enrollment be wrapped up by August 1. "I'm very goal oriented," explains Evelyn, "and I'm not going to miss my goal." A round of urgent phone calls ensued. They called the investigator; he was 100 percent on board and could see the patient earlier. They spoke to the monitor, who got in touch with the patient's daughter. The patient, an elderly man, was at a shopping mall, but without a phone—not an uncommon situation in that era. And his daughter didn't have a car.

Evelyn was resolute: "We sent a car service to pick up the daughter, to go to the mall to get the guy." They hit the deadline. The last number went on the tally board. Done. "You've got to drive the process," was Evelyn's favorite catchphrase. "You've got to ride 'em like a mule! Ride 'em like a mule!"

In the horse race against Genentech, it was a winning strategy. Eyetech recruited 578 patients in North America and 612 internationally. Everybody was invested in their success—the sites, the doctors, and especially, the patients. "We enrolled the whole thing in nine months," exalts Tony. "It was extraordinary."

$100 MILLION IS NOT ACADEMIC

When David considered the direction his career was taking, there were definitely some big upsides to being a professor, particularly as he had advanced to chairman of the ophthalmology department in 2000. Tenure being paramount. "The guy before me at NYU, as the chair, he was like eighty years old," says David, rekindling a spark from his former life. "I'm thinking, this could be permanent employment for forty years if I was lucky." For someone newly immersed in the world of risk assessment, academia wasn't even on the spectrum of hazardous occupations; the ivory tower provided the ultimate safe haven. In finance lingo, David's work streams were thoroughly diversified. "I was trying to keep them both going," David claims, referring to his academic and business pursuits. He figured if the drug didn't work, he could always fall back on teaching. As a resident, he never considered anything but a career in academia. But now, he was being seduced by a whole new sensation, something entirely absent in the scholarly world—speed. He felt invigorated by the pace of biotech.

For years, David's dalliance with drug development was indeed academic. It largely involved explaining the lab work of Tony and his cohort to knowledgeable audiences. Then, following Genentech's rejection, it involved searching through volumes of published research material to find other similarly promising molecules. His dean at NYU, Bob Glickman, was fine with David's extracurricular pursuits. "I would go three or more days a week to NYU," explains David about his time commitment, "or see patients and do administrative stuff, and at noon, I'd go to the Eyetech offices in Midtown." He was very busy but breezing along.

Following the culmination of the Series C financing, there was a sea change. Making waves on Wall Street had a ripple effect on NYU's campus in Greenwich Village. Glickman informed David, "Look, I'm getting people on my board who read in *Crain's New York Business* about this gigantic fundraising." The reactions the dean received weren't positive. "They're saying that guy's your department chairman; how can he do both?" In

Glickman's view, David was a victim of his own success. "You've raised too much money." In the dean's mind, the answer to this dilemma was to forgo the acclamation rather than the actual cash. "I'm fine if you work with the company," he said to David, but his ultimatum was "you can't be CEO and department chairman."

Keeping his academic hat on, David resolved to deal with this situation semantically. "I tried to figure out other titles," he recollects. "I saw at Yahoo! they called the CEO, chief Yahoo, not CEO. So, I came to the dean the next day and said, 'I could be chief eye officer?' Still CEO." It didn't fly. Instead, the pair resolved that David could take a sabbatical for a year. Once again, academia delivered a risk-averse future.

Tony found himself in an identical position at Harvard. "I did the same thing," he recounts. "I went to my dean, and I was able to get a one-year sabbatical, although we never called it that." Ever a true scientist, his was an empirical decision process: "I knew that in a one-year time period we would get our initial data." If he clearly saw the drug was doing something, then he could cut the cord to academia and go full time into the biotech business. Meanwhile, Tony split his attention between Boston and New York: "I was on the air shuttle and Amtrak all the time."

Samir had been in a state of flux, spending up to four days per week in New York. But once the large trial was underway, he moved from Chicago to fully assume his role as chief of clinical and commercial strategy. He was constantly in David's ear, providing advice from his perspective as an outstanding clinician.

Having three eye doctors deeply engaged in the daily activities of a biotech start-up was unprecedented. But they were wise enough to recognize their need for someone experienced in the business minutiae.

"Out of the blue, I got a call about this amazing company," remembers Glenn Sblendorio, "from a recruiter at Heidrick & Struggles." After meeting with Marty, John, and David, he wound up at 666 Fifth Avenue, which despite its location was underwhelming and overcrowded. "I walked into an office, maybe it was two thousand square feet." He noted that

David's shared office was multifunctional: "It was also the conference room and the team room; he had a couch in there." Tasked with building the organization, Glenn found it easy to envisage progress, particularly given where he had already been.

In 1980, with an undergraduate degree in accounting and a CPA, Glenn started at Roche in its audit group. But rather than keeping his head down counting beans, he quickly began ruffling feathers. At the time, Roche was transforming itself from a motley collection of regional companies into a global juggernaut. Glenn's analysis of how Roche spent its capital got on the radar of some very senior people. "I rose pretty quickly. And I was one of the first folks to start to travel internationally," he says about his early career. "I met the people in Basel." This included bigwigs like the CFO Henry Meyer, who worked closely with CEOs Fritz Gerber and Irwin Lerner to reshape the corporation. Eventually, Glenn moved to Switzerland and worked there for Amgen. While there, he received another intriguing call from a recruiter, who told him about an opportunity with an entertainment company. Despite Glenn responding that he sells drugs, not video games, the recruiter persisted, emphasizing Glenn's deep licensing experience. The conversation led to Glenn becoming the global CFO for Sony's PlayStation, just in time for the gaming platform's launch.

After four years of thrills in the gaming world, Glenn realized he missed his former life. "I really did love pharmaceuticals, and I loved healthcare. The end result, that you're helping patients," he reflects, "I had to get back to that." While powering along his unusual career trajectory, Glenn also managed to acquire an MBA in finance. With a former Roche colleague from Switzerland, Clive Meanwell, he began working in venture capital and cofounded the Medicines Company. *Forbes* repeatedly ranked the biotech disruptor a top innovator for its unique focus on reviving drugs that, due to technicalities, had failed FDA trials and then finding new applications for them—dubbed a "Lazarus strategy" by the publication. For Glenn, the Medicines Company expanded his financial horizons: "I got to know the banking community, got to know the venture community." When the Medicines Company went public and started zeroing in on cardiovascular treatments, Glenn found himself restless again. That's when he received the timely call from Heidrick & Struggles. As a kid, Glenn had wheeled his blind grandmother about. His grandfather, too, had difficulty seeing. "They had macular degeneration," he explains, "but we didn't realize it."

PFIZER ON ICE

Nobody needed 20/20 vision to see that Eyetech had outgrown its digs on Fifth Avenue. People were literally working on top of each other. The search for more space led to an entirely different section of Manhattan. Although lacking the gleaming towers in the heart of the island, the aging, set-back buildings of the Garment District (a wedding cake–like architectural style once mandated to let more light reach the floor of the metropolis but long abandoned) offered close proximity to Penn Station, which appealed greatly to the numerous New Jerseyites on staff. Globalization in the latter part of the twentieth century had done much to empty out this formerly bustling light manufacturing zone. Where once it was common to witness trolleys laden with blouses and jackets dangling from coat hangers rumble along the sidewalks forming textile traffic jams, now a strange absence of activity seeped out of the largely vacant loading bays lining the streets. Fashion designers stayed, now using software to digitally assemble their lines. But the rows and rows of cutting and sewing machines that used to viscerally and noisily piece together their creations on the lower floors beneath their studios were gone, replaced by sweatshops in Asia and Latin America.

SoHo in lower Manhattan had already gone through a similar transition. A generation earlier, artists had replaced garment factories and fabric warehouses. When the Loft Law legalized their residence in formerly industrial spaces in 1981, gentrification quickly followed. But after the recession in the early 1990s and the dot-com crash in 2000, landlords in the Garment District were unsure their future would mirror the past, and the promising encroachment of Silicon Alley appeared to have reached a dead end. All of which created a favorable rental market for the extremely cashed-up Eyetech.

"We moved down to Thirty-Seventh Street and did a kind of high-tech office," Glenn recounts, describing the new environment on the sixteenth floor of the industrial building they occupied. "We made it cool. Really cool. We had all these tall, open ceilings, and everyone was in the hallways all the time. The day-to-day was...it was always crazy."

With the need for office space resolved—at least for the time being—there was another pressing issue, involving a very different concept of space: how to continue to develop, and then commercialize the drug at a global scale. "We got advanced enough where we needed a partner," explains David about the idea of a licensing deal. "We couldn't do ex-US ourself. We were too small."

The quest for an ex-US partner began around the same time as the recruitment effort got underway but took on new urgency after the move to the Garment District. Originally, Eyetech courted the New Jersey–based Pharmacia. In David's view, "Pharmacia was the natural partner; they were really into ophthalmology." Discussions had reached as far as a term sheet. As a promising young company, Eyetech also evidently had many other term sheets from major pharma companies in hand, but Pharmacia was the frontrunner. "Everything was great," David recounts. "Then we wake up one day and we see Pfizer bought them. We're like, oh my God! This got messed up."

Pfizer, the world's biggest drug company, paid $60 billion for Pharmacia, adding significantly to its cancer-fighting repertoire while augmenting its already broad range of cardiac therapies. Given that Pfizer had recently also swallowed Warner-Lambert for $115 billion, it was easy to imagine the fledgling ophthalmology start-up getting completely lost in the churn. However, Pharmacia considered its potential deal with Eyetech to be so significant, it had apparently instituted a "carve out" provision in its sale to Pfizer to allow it to continue with Eyetech while undergoing all the regulatory reviews such huge transactions must endure before receiving FTC approval.

It's good to feel like a favorite child in a soon-to-be extended family. But on the other hand, why not just cozy up to the big new daddy? If Eyetech could effectively leverage Pfizer's massive size, that would be a whole other scenario. David felt that Pfizer was "the Harvard of pharma at the time. They were in New York." He sums it up, "I kind of liked them."

And with all the term sheets Eyetech had gathered, David consulted with his chief outside lawyer, David Redlick. What if they could turn the tables and play the pharma giants against each other? The little company may have a negotiating advantage, despite its size. So they got a term sheet from Pfizer, too. The way they saw it, with Pharmacia under its wing, Pfizer was now interested in ophthalmology as well.

In what was an unusual business strategy. David Redlick's team drafted contracts simultaneously for all three finalist pharma companies. Essentially, with the deals on the table being very similar in nature, Eyetech wanted to conclude the process quickly—to keep its momentum. Now, the race was on. For this maneuver to work, Eyetech needed to be transparent about all its conversations. "We told them all upfront. It was pretty aggressive," says David about his desire to instill a sense of rivalry among the big firms. "Whoever signed the contract first would win the deal. And every time someone started fighting us on stuff, we'd say, 'Look, we're going to spend more time with someone else ahead of you.'"

The scheme worked. Indeed, so well, it provoked Henry McKinnell, Pfizer's CEO, to ask his head of business development, "Who are these guys?" To which he received the answer, "They're the biggest biotech firm in the Garment District." This claim to fame still didn't mean Eyetech was ready to accommodate Pfizer's team when they paid a visit to conduct their due diligence. The large swarm of visitors forced the Eyetech folks to scramble at the last minute and rent extra chairs to seat everyone.

"Then, I remember, Pfizer came up with a list of about twenty things,"

David recounts. He then consulted his board member Damion Wicker: "He said, 'Don't talk to them for four days.' I'm like, 'How can you do that? They're Pfizer!'" Despite having to ignore tons of emails and phone calls, which he found extremely difficult, David followed the advice: "We totally blew them off. And then finally, I come into the office, and I see eight of them just standing outside the door. Just showed up. And they said, 'We cave,' and 'Let's just get this done as soon as possible; whatever, all the points we give into.'" Bringing this to mind still feels very satisfying to David: "It was very effective to basically, I guess 'ghost' them is what they call it now. We used to call it 'icing.' We iced them."

But there was one sticking point. An Eyetech board member noticed that the tiny European island nation of Malta was paying a slightly lower royalty than its bigger neighbors. This struck him as a potential loophole, which needed to be closed. The head of Pfizer's business development team couldn't believe this could possibly be a deal-breaker. He incredulously told David, "You have one board member who thinks Pfizer is going to take the potential liability and public relations disaster of a picture of their reps flying to Malta, stocking up with drugs in their suitcase, and selling them in France and Italy to save 2 percent on the royalty. Is that what the issue is?" David assured him: "Yes, that's the issue." He looked at David and replied, "Okay. We can fix this." Then he continued, "I would like to meet that board member. But only once."

With the issue resolved and a chill in the air, *The Wall Street Journal* immediately reported the news on December 18, 2002, laying bare the deal details: "Pfizer will make initial payments of $100 million, with $195 million in possible milestone payments, based on gaining regulatory approvals." Not only would Pfizer "pay for the majority of the development costs for the drug," but Eyetech also had "the potential to receive up to $450 million in additional milestone payments, based on successful commercialization and sales levels." With Eyetech keeping all US rights and significant ex-US royalties, it was one of the two largest ex-US partnership deals between biotech and pharma done to date.

TRUE PARTNERS

If ever there was a time of relative calm for Eyetech, it was the year following the Pfizer deal. Injecting the eyes of hundreds of patients around the world with a novel drug was hardly routine, and the result was unpredictable, even if it seemed highly favorable. But this is exactly what David and his team had set out to do. While there were constantly things to attend to, David could carve out the time to take care of the most important event in his life—his wedding.

Having met in the Hamptons, Maria and David thought it fitting to tie the knot there. However, true to form, David couldn't resist adding a subtle element of risk: a beach wedding late in the year. "We got super lucky," he says of their big day. "It was seventy degrees."

On November 1, at Westhampton Beach, on the southern shore of New York's Long Island, in front of 120 guests, David and Maria took their vows. The ceremony was conducted by a rabbi and a priest. It was by all accounts spectacular. "We sat on the beach, with no jackets," remembers Katherine. "It was the most picture-perfect, beautiful day. They had a beautiful, beautiful wedding."

Chapter 7

GOING PUBLIC

"You've got to do this!" David insisted Evelyn join him on a private jet trip to Boston for a roadshow. "When you get up there, make sure you go to the bathroom," Evelyn recalls being coaxed by her boss. "They've got everything you can think of."

In the sprint toward the company's initial public offering, private jets became the mode of transport du jour. How else could you hit three or more cities in a single day to pitch to twenty different investors? No crazy lines at airport security. No delays. No other passengers. Evelyn accepted. With one condition: Loni and Denis had to come along, too. "If they don't get to go on the private jet," Evelyn pleaded, "I won't be able to work in peace!"

On board, Evelyn was impressed: "It was awesome. The bathroom's got wood paneling. And I got to fly in the jump seat with the pilot when they were landing." But on this trip, like all the other legs of the nearly two weeks of continuous private air travel for the senior executive team, the most amazing thing wasn't the bathroom. It was the food. Forget commercial airline meals, blanched of all flavor. "On those trips," Evelyn explains, "whatever city you went to, whatever food you wanted, you would tell the flight attendants, and they would order it from any place you wanted in that city. And when you got back to the plane, the food would be on the plane. And David knows restaurants everywhere. David had a whole list."

In Boston, it was pasta from David's old standby during his days there with Tony: the Daily Catch in the North End, famous for its squid-ink linguine served in iron skillets. "It was always great food," David reminisces, "wherever *it* was. Deep-dish pizza, Chicago; ribs, St. Louis; La Taqueria, Mexican, San Francisco; Joe's Stone Crab, Miami Beach; BBQ, Atlanta. We would find a hole in the wall or the best rib place in Kansas City, and we would eat there, or they would bring it on the plane."

Glenn, a constant companion on the journey to pitch investors, says of David, "His number one passion is food." Speak to anyone involved with Eyetech, and the conversation ultimately leads to the same flavorful subject. An army may march on its stomach; at Eyetech the driving force was taste buds. Long before Uber Eats and scores of dining apps converged on people's phones, David captured his team's attention with his unrelenting pursuit of captivating cuisines.

Growing up on Long Island, more famous for suburban conformity than culinary diversity, was limiting. "I didn't know what was out there," David reflects. "Then I went to college, saw more ethnic diversity and food that was exciting." His keen interest in spice developed during his residency at Johns Hopkins, exploring Baltimore restaurants with Sumit Nanda, a fellow resident whose family was from India and craved familiar flavors from his ancestral homeland. But David's palate really kicked into high gear when he joined forces with Samir. "He had a very deep passion," David says of his friend. "It was a common interest. Traveling so much around the world with him is really what brought that out the most."

The duo became inseparable on the Association of University Professors of Ophthalmology (AUPO) circuit when Samir was residency director at the University of Chicago and David at the Manhattan Eye and Ear Infirmary. Travel was nearly constant. "We were at many meetings internationally together," David reminisces. "I've definitely traveled with Samir more than anybody in my life. I wouldn't be surprised if we traveled to more than fifty or sixty countries." As they traversed the globe, climbing ever higher up the Scoville scale for heat became an unending challenge, uncovering and sampling the hottest dish their Mount Everest.

Samir remembers an early AUPO meeting in the Arizona desert as a watershed moment. This gathering of chairpeople and residency directors presented a great opportunity to raise interest in the pair's burgeoning drug research, but the schedule had a large hole in it. David, after learning that the Grand Canyon was within driving distance, decided that visiting the world's most famous chasm would be the ideal way to fill the void. Samir declined David's invitation to join him. He'd already seen it once. However, at four o'clock the following morning, there was a pounding on Samir's hotel room door. Alarmed, Samir thought it was a fire. In a panic, he rushed to the door, only to find David with two cups of coffee. "You know what? It's only four hours away, the Grand Canyon," David coaxed. "I got coffee for you. You don't have to do anything. The car's running, and it's dark outside still."

With considerable restraint, Samir managed not to punch his eager friend and instead reminded him, "We have a thing at four o'clock this afternoon."

Samir was learning that tenacity was one of his friend's defining characteristics. David was undeterred: "Can you just do me a favor? Can you get in the backseat and just fall asleep? I want to do all the driving." As became habitual in their relationship, David's insistence led to Samir's relenting. "It's so persistent," Samir explains, "that you have to give in. Because if you don't, just the fight itself will raise your blood pressure to an enormous extent."

It's hard to imagine that seeing the Grand Canyon was a nonevent. But for David, a quick glimpse leaning over a guardrail was sufficient. He instantly got the picture (without needing to take one). And to Samir's exasperation, no sooner had they got out of the car than they were back on the road returning to the AUPO meeting. He fumed, "You made me do this for four hours each way?"

David was contrite: "I'm going to definitely make this up. Wait till you see."

After the meeting, David approached the concierge at the hotel and asked her, "What is your favorite Mexican food here?" She volunteered a restaurant name. David continued, "What's your second favorite?" After she named another place, David persevered. "What's the third favorite?" By this stage, the woman was rattled. The eye doctor explained he wasn't trying to be a belligerent guest; he just desired to dive deeper. "I don't want to know what you tell the people here at the Biltmore. I want to know where *you* go with your friends, where you'd not send people—that's *really* authentic." In the days before Google, Yelp, ChatGPT, and the multitude of online diner reviews and apps, David honed this approach to break through the protective crust concierges developed to shield tourists from spicy food that would overwhelm their fragile palates. Eventually, the woman opened up: There was a place, right at the edge of town, Los Dos Molinos, named after a pair of antique chili grinders, heirlooms of the owners. In the years since David and Samir's first visit, the small family restaurant has become widely respected, sprouting a more central sister location. On its menu it warns wary diners, "Food is spicy! You order it. You own it." And, "I am sorry, we do not provide mild sauce. I do not know how to make it 'Mild.'"

David and Samir arrived at Los Dos Molinos to find a huge line outside for an inside table. They weren't the only ones keen to savor the spiciest food in Phoenix. A two-hour wait wasn't something the doctors had counted on. David compensated for his complete lack of patience by cranking up his ingenuity and asking a server if they could get takeout. Not a problem, he was assured. Immediately, David rattled off an order for about ten items. This technique, best described as "reverse omakase," furnishes a tasting menu absent the discretion of the chef but complete with full-size servings. Not only does this method provide the opportunity to sample a broad swath of the selections on offer, but the diversity reduces the chance a single unappealing choice will ruin a meal (especially helpful when a return visit is unlikely). Plus, it also has the side effect of winning favor with the establishment due to the swollen size of the resulting check. This unintended benefit of David's signature request style has earned him a glowing reputation at dining premises of all sizes and stripes around the planet, from roadside shacks to white linen restaurants with multiple Michelin stars.

Successful at leapfrogging the line, David then conducted a little sneaky furniture rearranging, grabbing two chairs and a table in the courtyard in front of Los Dos Molinos and hiding them behind a tree and a small wall. "Okay, now we can start eating," David declared, remaining aloof to the attention he'd drawn from the nearby hungry crowd still waiting. His efforts were well rewarded. "I'm telling you," Samir insists, "it was the bloody spiciest thing you ever had. I'm Indian; I can eat really spicy food!"

Once David has successfully unearthed culinary gold, he stops prospecting and digs in. As David sees it, "Why experiment when you find perfection?" This can mean eating repeatedly in the same establishment the entire time he's in a city. Samir recalls adhering to this with David in Rio de Janeiro at Fogo de Chão, the churrascaria which ultimately became an international chain. "We would go to this same place every single day," Samir says of their visit. "Lunch and dinner, lunch and dinner, lunch and dinner. It was the same thing every single day. Picanha and special cheese." In Rome, the sole venue was La Mani in Pasta, in the hip neighborhood of Trastevere. "David likes it so much," Samir recalls. "He would order five or six helpings for two people with massive, massive plates. It's a very tiny place; we got to know the owner so David could sit right next to the kitchen window." Samir maintains David's infatuation doesn't diminish over time: "Subsequently through all his other companies, he must have gone there, including family vacations, at least forty-five to fifty times."

David acknowledges his obsession: "My kids will say there's only one restaurant in Rome because we would eat lunch and dinner at La Mani in Pasta four days in a row, eight meals. But if I took you there, you'd see why." Repetitive dining has benefits. "We were like royalty there. They'd hug us and kiss us, even though they couldn't even speak English."

SO MANY PLACES TO EAT, SO LITTLE TIME. BUT SO MUCH MONEY ON THE TABLE!

Of course, recurring visits to a restaurant can only happen during prolonged stays in a city. With the rapid turnaround time of the travel for investment pitching, David perfected another patience hack. "This is the greatest trick in the world," Samir recalls. "Wherever he goes, whenever at a restaurant, whenever he needs food, he says, 'We have to go to the airport.'" The impact is immediate and profound, overcoming any language barriers. "David learned that whenever you use the word *airport*, they'll rush whatever it is and anything else you tell them."

The private jet spree to raise money for the IPO was the perfect synthesis of David's roving appetite and unrelenting urgency. With the food often greeting the team on the plane, the runway became the restaurant. David explains this was more than a matter of convenience: "When you've given fifteen lectures a day in three cities and you're exhausted, it's something you look forward to, kind of a motivating force in many ways." But there was one incident on board that had stomachs churning, and not in a good way.

The team was in Texas, dashing to three cities in a day in a Gulfstream V, a spacious and luxurious jet in the upper echelon of private aircraft at the time. "All of sudden, the plane went down hard. It just did a tremendous nosedive. Took our breath away, our stomachs away," David recalls. "We all thought the plane was crashing." It turns out, not even the pilot was aware of what was happening. "It actually was an automated evasive maneuver." He elaborates, "What happened was a little, tiny plane without a beacon—their beacon was broken, they shouldn't have been flying—showed up in the clouds. It was like an unregistered plane. And the jet was so sophisticated that, without the pilot even knowing, it just did a nosedive. And obviously saved our lives."

David and his intrepid crew were lucky in another way, too. Although the expediency of using private jets was clear to his investors, some of them were giving him a hard time about flying in a top-of-the-line aircraft.

"Why don't you just spend half and get a lesser plane?" they asked him. Fortunately, his general counsel held firm and said, "No, no, no, we're going to go spend it. You've got to be about safety." David ruminates, "Think about it. If it was a lesser plane, without that advanced detection system, we might've crashed." Not only would lives have been lost, but all the investors' money would have been gone, too. Today, David only flies commercial, preferably on the biggest plane possible. What counts is the experience of the pilot. The more senior, the better.

Despite the risks, David's approach clearly worked. With over 120 pitches delivered to investors across two continents, the results speak for themselves. "Ninety-nine percent of the places we went to pitch put an order in for shares," David proudly recalls. His charisma bolstered the appeal—investors must have felt their money was in good hands—but the clear science and the size of the unmet medical need drove the fundraising. In backing Eyetech, Wall Street showed it had greater foresight than Big Pharma. Also, having someone like Glenn on board, who understood the workings of Wall Street, was key to the company's success. Knowing exactly who to pitch to is vital, particularly when time is in short supply. Jetting about the country was grounded in diligent footwork.

Having raised a lot of capital earlier in his career, Glenn had relationships with Morgan Stanley and Merrill Lynch. "I worked a lot with those guys," he says looking back. "We could get a meeting with anybody, and we met with every single bank." But in those pre–Dodd Frank days, Glenn maintains, the key person to impress was the analyst. "The Wall Street analyst got paid based on trading activity. The analyst could sit in the same room as the bankers." Following the financial crisis of 2007 and 2008, the legislation built a wall between banks' research and trading operations, ending that cozy arrangement. "Back then it was all about getting the analyst, the best analyst. So, David and I, we had two favorites: Steve Harr who was at Morgan Stanley and Eric Ende at Merrill Lynch. Those were the two guys to get because they had the best client list."

Once more, little Eyetech found itself playing two giants against each other. Both investment banks wanted to be "on the left side of the book," leading the underwriting process, gathering orders from institutional investors—a process known as "building the book"—responsible for driving the demand for shares, setting their price, and arranging allocation. Naturally, being the primary underwriter garners a bigger payoff than simply joining the syndicate of investors. For a while, Glenn favored Merrill Lynch, who went out of their way to woo Eyetech. But in the end, Glenn says, "Morgan Stanley came on really strong, made a lot of appropriate promises about coverage, meeting schedules, and got their number two guy involved who delivered us Steve Harr." That sealed the deal. Morgan Stanley got the top slot, but Merrill Lynch, CS First Boston, and Bear Stearns were also along for the ride.

It was a hell of a ride, beyond the comfort of the jet and the food. Not only did every pitch barring one succeed in attracting investment, but the journey ended with a subscription level that was an astounding thirty times over the actual available offering. Investor appetite was so great that securing just a tiny piece of the action was an achievement but often left financiers grumbling, hungry for more.

After frantically zooming around Europe and the US for two weeks, the big day loomed. Morgan Stanley set the stock price on January 29, 2004: 6.5 million common shares under the EYET symbol would be available on the NASDAQ stock market at the start of the next day for twenty-one dollars per share, with a total value of $157 million (including the additional 15 percent of "greenshoe" shares the underwriter reserved for price stabilization but not those under "lock-up" retained by the founders and initial investors). It was a tense moment in the Biotech world. The window on Biotech IPOs had been shut for a while, and investors were wondering what effect prying it open would have. The Eyetech IPO was viewed as a barometer for the entire industry. Could the success of the start-up behind closed doors be replicated on the worldwide stage of capital markets?

Eyetech was the first biotech IPO of 2004. Following a dismal environment in the fourth quarter of the previous year, its performance was closely scrutinized. Commentators had been eagerly anticipating a turnaround in the market. As early as August 2003, *The Wall Street Journal* ran a story titled "Biotech Industry Edges Toward IPO Boomlet." Still, that reversal of fortune had yet to occur. Just a month before going public, the publication proclaimed, "In the sagging market for biotechnology-company IPOs, all eyes are on Eyetech Pharmaceuticals Inc." and noted that for recent offerings, "investors' reaction to the flurry of deals has been less than enthusiastic."

When David and the Eyetech team arrived at the NASDAQ building in Times Square to ring the opening bell for the exchange at nine thirty in the morning on Friday, January 30, they were confident but on edge. "We knew it was going to be strong," says Glenn, thinking back on the anticipation, "[but] we didn't know how good the IPO was going to be." It didn't take long to find out. As soon as David's signature unfurled on the electronic display behind the launch podium, trading was brisk. By the end of the day, the stock price had leaped an astonishing 54 percent, soaring $11.40 to close at $32.40. Eyetech's logo lit up the giant cylindrical LED screen that wrapped around the exchange's building, the seven-story tall focal point of Times Square. Eyetech dominated the crossroads of the world! It was the biggest-ever first-day increase for a biotech company. In a mere three years, ten months, and twenty-one days, Eyetech had gone from an idea to a public company valued at $926.8 million.

After a ton of photo ops with the entire company in and outside the NASDAQ building, all that was left to do was to prove Eyetech was really worth that much.

WORKING HARD, PLAYING HARD

Normally, when you go from being valued at a theoretical $436 million in the morning to just shy of a verified $1 billion that same afternoon, some serious celebration is in order. Following the close of trading, the Eyetech team enjoyed a large cake decorated with its logo in frosting and a few rounds of champagne in the NASDAQ offices. Glasses clinked; congratulations were shared; but that was it. They were exhausted from the hectic airborne roadshow of the preceding weeks and the huge adrenaline rush of the day. Being a company led by medical professionals, they appreciated their physical limitations. Still, it was an unusually subdued finale. Although not on display that day, as a true New York company, Eyetech was as proud of its party ethic as much as its work ethic. Indeed, in its brief existence, Eyetech had garnered a reputation in ophthalmological circles for throwing the hottest ticket in town whenever eye doctors and their ilk assembled en masse.

* * *

At the Academy of Ophthalmology's annual gathering in Anaheim the previous November, the lucky five hundred well-dressed partygoers who got past the tight security—with guards sporting earpieces—were set to experience something sensational. Three massive ballrooms, bedecked with ice sculptures surrounded by ten thousand white roses and lilies, hosted a smorgasbord of enticing cuisines. "That was the best party I've ever thrown," remembers Evelyn (officially VP of clinical development, unofficially president of party planning). "It was just spectacular. I had to pay the band extra to keep playing and not shut down at ten o'clock because people refused to stop dancing."

While the night is long remembered for its extended dance floor antics, the all-out celebration followed the release of initial Phase 3 trial data to a large number of the doctors conducting the tests. Indeed, the festivities were part of an orchestrated exercise in building Eyetech's corporate brand prior to launching its drug. The eagerly anticipated results were part of a carefully choreographed performance at the AAO, with Judah Folkman delivering the keynote address. His presence solidified the decade of research since VEGF was detected in the retina. Fittingly, the night's festivities were taking place just a few miles down the Pacific coast from where David and Tony first daydreamed about a therapeutic approach to macular degeneration inspired by Folkman's work, at the last AAO meeting held in Anaheim, twelve years earlier.

The trial results stirred up the celebratory mood. Eyetech demonstrated patients receiving Macugen had a significantly reduced rate of vision loss compared to those in the control group. About 70 percent of patients treated with Macugen maintained their vision (defined as losing fewer than three lines of visual acuity on an eye chart over one year). For those in the control group, the vision loss was far greater. Finally, eye doctors would have some good news to tell their suffering patients.

Of course, the AAO was a marquee event, but the numerous milestones along Eyetech's journey sparked outbursts of festivity. "We were forever having some type of celebration," asserts Evelyn. There were boat rides at ARVO's annual meetings in Fort Lauderdale and one in New York following the success of the Series C fundraising. One extra sparkly holiday party coincided with the Pfizer partnership.

To paint an accurate portrait of the company's social side, it's vital to step away from strobe lighting and mirror balls. David supported a wide variety of team-building activities. In addition to holding company picnics in Central Park, Eyetech joined a softball league based there and played weekly games against other New York firms with David as shortstop. "You've got to develop a culture and do things," exhorts David, "whether it be retreats, softball teams, or dinners that bring people together." A prescription that rings even truer in the era of hybrid work.

Running was also a favorite. Having competed five times in both the New York and Boston marathons, David was eager to sponsor road races, typically ten-kilometer events around the park. This included a New York marathon, chaperoning a young, blind athlete from Australia in conjunction with Achilles International, an organization dedicated to helping people with disabilities engage in physical activities. David was supposed to use a short rope to guide her through the throngs of runners. "She was so fast," David chuckles. "We all had trouble keeping up with her." Sporting the advantage of youth, it became a case of the blind leading the sighted.

Beyond conventional gatherings and sporting events, Evelyn notes there was one unusual activity David was especially fond of: "He would make everybody go to laser tag in Times Square." With Macugen poised to replace zapping eyeballs in doctor's offices around the world, could David have been subconsciously holding on for one last flash of excitement?

* * *

Now a public company, Eyetech's value was continuously calibrated in the stock market. But this measure fails to appreciate the inherent worth of its culture. Twenty years later, many of its employees and officers recall working there as one of the greatest experiences in their lives. While it's a pity capitalism doesn't factor worker happiness in its metrics, regardless of how the company's ethos was assessed, the shine never dimmed on Eyetech in the financial world. "I'd go to banking conferences and was good friends with the Merrill Lynch guys," Glenn recounts. "And I'll never forget, in 2004—and this is before the drug was launched—they talked about us as the 'number one company on Wall Street.'"

In many ways, this was due to Eyetech's skillful navigation of the confluence between the different flows of medical research and finance. Because market conditions were so poor at the end of 2003, the company needed to build confidence by releasing its Phase 3 data before going public. "The Phase 3 data was enough to get investors there," David says about the timing. "And obviously, the venture investors want liquidity; they want to do an IPO. So we opened the market, and it was a tough market." By comparison, he says, "There are other times where preclinical companies, before even putting a drug in humans, can go public, when there are frothy markets."

It's a testament to how much Eyetech changed market sentiment that just a few months after the initial IPO, they could mount a secondary offering. In late May, the lock-up period for a large number of shares was terminated early, and they were sold for $38.50 per share, allowing the initial investors to take advantage of the company's momentum, at an 83 percent premium. Typically, second offerings have a slightly detrimental impact on a company's stock price. Usually, there's about a 10 percent dip during the week of the offering's roadshow, as investors sense a share dilution coming or perceive that the need for cash is an indication something is wrong at the company. But everything at Eyetech was going extremely well. The roadshow coincided with positive data from the Phase 2 trial of Macugen for DME, and even more significantly, that month Eyetech had filed for FDA approval for treating wet AMD. But despite the positive momentum of the company, David was still prepared for Eyetech's price to go down.

David's team was busy doing twelve meetings a day with investors in New York when a strange thing happened. "It was about ten in the morning; we're in an elevator about to go up and pitch," he says of the moment. "And Loni says to me, 'Oh my God! Our stock just went up 20 percent!' I'm like, 'That's impossible. It should be going down.'" David explains how this financial anomaly occurred: "By pure coincidence, the FDA, on their website, just announced that they were calling an early advisory meeting for our drug." This was an opportunity for the agency's experts to garner outside expertise. David continues, "Which was a very bullish sign. Usually, it could be nine months later. The FDA said, 'Oh, we're going to do it in four months.' So they accelerated the data meeting of the advisory panel, and the street looked at that as a gigantic sign that the FDA was going to approve it. And it made our stock price go way up during the secondary roadshow. Which never happens!"

SUMMER SCHOOL IS NOT COOL

"I remember spending the whole summer studying for it," David says about appearing before the FDA advisory panel. After years of being a professor, he felt like he was reliving his student day—"like studying for your medical boards," he recalls. To ease the ordeal, one of his board members suggested hiring a tutor. The man he had in mind was Thomas Fleming, from the University of Washington in Seattle, regarded as one of the world's greatest biotech and pharma biostatisticians. This maneuver had two benefits. First, it ensured they were getting the best advice possible. The second was more surreptitious. After being on scores of FDA advisory panels, Fleming earned a reputation, acknowledged by David, for "taking drugs out [of consideration] because he's so smart statistically." Although advisory panels don't have the final say in approving a drug—that lies with the FDA itself—their recommendations carry weight, often causing considerable delays in drugs reaching the market. "You don't want him on the panel," David continues half-jokingly. "So if you make him a consultant, you contaminate him! But more importantly, he prepares you so well for the panel."

Just as toxins can become vaccines, Eyetech felt Fleming's sting before building immunity. "I remember the first time we met him; we were at a long table, and everybody introduced themselves, and he said, 'I'm Wiley Chambers, the head of the FDA' instead of saying, 'I'm Tom Fleming.' And then he just destroyed us." David recounts Tom Fleming's roleplaying, "He asked us questions, millions of questions; we'd all have headaches after spending time with this guy. We spent days and days and days with him, and he'd find something with statistics, 'Well, why did this happen? Does this mean this?'" Fleming's approach was relentless; even the most esteemed ophthalmologists advising Eyetech weren't spared. "We had people like Don D'Amico, chairman at Cornell, who was there, and he just would destroy him," David recounts, reflecting on the intense interrogation. "D'Amico said, 'I've never been questioned like that in my life.' People were actually scared, overwhelmed, exhausted."

Fleming's fusillades had a purpose. "The beauty," David reflects, "is he would break you down. It was just grueling, but then, he would give you the answers why. It was the greatest preparation in the world. When we went into the FDA advisory panel, you kind of felt like nobody could hurt you because Tom Fleming had thought of everything and challenged you, and he then gave you the answers. And there, frankly, was no one as difficult or tough."

The second ally who helped Eyetech prep for the big test on August 27 was Pfizer. No stranger to the ordeal, the pharma giant put its vast resources in action. After all, Macugen was their potential billion-dollar baby, too. Where Pfizer shone was its mastery of visual presentation. "For any possible question that could be asked, there was a slide," David explains, "like thirty-five thousand slides. It was insane. It was an army." Images for every conceivable situation—showing the drug mechanism, its effectiveness and safety, plus all manner of statistical analysis—were at the ready. For David, the challenge was how to take command. What good are all those troops if they're not obeying your orders? "I mean," David explains, "if someone asks you a question, how do you know what slide to look at?"

Pfizer had a solution up its sleeve. A device the size of a small alarm clock, a little monitor, sat on the stand in front of David, displaying the number of the slide to bring up. But there was one catch: When the panel of experts facing David asked a question, David had to play for time and repeat it, buying a precious few seconds so Pfizer's team of technicians and Matt Feinsod from Eyetech—hiding out of sight in a space off the main, drab, windowless room—could search through their library and relay the number of the slide to him. When the digits flashed before him, David would look up and say, "Could I please have slide 11,483?" This would then be displayed on the screen for everyone in the room to see. To this day, David doesn't know how the team worked so quickly, but it helped him impress the panel: "It gave the impression to the audience that I had memorized all thirty-five thousand slides, that I knew at the tip of my tongue which slide that data was on." This sleight of hand worked. David's apparent photographic memory evidently impressed the members of the advisory panel, giving the FDA comfort that the Eyetech team understood the data so meticulously and had studied it so thoroughly that they knew it by heart.

After the arduous preparation, the meeting went well. It even began with a softball question from a panel member, a professor of ethics at the University of Texas, who asked, since the data was so good, why didn't Eyetech stop its trial early for ethical reasons? This allowed David to explain that the trial needed to continue to ensure it reached a statistically valid benchmark.

Undoubtedly the most effective moment during the advisory meeting, however, had nothing to do with data. David asked a Californian friend for a favor. Steve Schwartz was an ophthalmologist and a professor at UCLA with a roster of celebrity patients. David asked, "Steve, can you bring a patient? A patient who can advocate for the drug." But when Schwartz showed up at the meeting, he was accompanied not by Hollywood royalty but by a frail old lady in her eighties, who was prepared to give her testimony completely unrehearsed. David recounts, "She gets up there, and she says how she was a Holocaust survivor, but going blind with macular degeneration was worse than being part of the Holocaust, and how Macugen helped her change her life." Everybody there was profoundly moved. "The whole room was just shaken. Nobody knew that was coming," remembers David. "The FDA reviewer who I was next to started crying."

With everything in order, the panel was unanimous in its support that the clinical data and the drug's efficacy outweighed any safety concerns. Approval was on track to occur before the end of the year.

A HOT MESS IN CANADA

Out of sight of the scrutiny of the advisory panel, there was one area where Eyetech was flailing—manufacturing. Before approving a drug, the FDA needs to make sure that a drug not only does what it's supposed to do in clinical trials and is safe, but it also needs to be ready for mass consumption. In bureaucratese, this is known as CMC: chemistry, manufacturing, and controls. "It was a disaster," Glenn says, summoning a memory that has weighed on his mind for two decades. "You've got to have three registration batches as part of your CMC package. And we had failure after failure in leading up to that."

Blame it on the butterfly effect—the idea embedded in chaos theory that small changes in one location can lead to dramatic, unpredictable consequences far away. But rather than the classic chaos theory example of the flap of insect wings in Brazil causing a tornado in Texas, in this case, F-117 Nighthawks delivering laser-guided bombs in Baghdad instigated a brain drain in Alberta, Canada. The Iraq War impacted oil prices around the globe, setting off fears of a shortage and triggering speculation in commodities markets. This anxiety-induced oil boom created a spike in demand for skilled workers right where Eyetech was attempting to produce the aptamer for Macugen in bulk, in a factory on the outskirts of Edmonton. "All the good scientists, even technicians," Glenn states with a trace of anguish, "were going to work for the oil companies who were paying double."

This set off a slew of problems. "I remember one time I got a call late in the night that a technician finished a batch and forgot to close the valve on the bottom, and the stuff leaked out the floor," complains Glenn. "It was that kind of nonsense." The solution was difficult. "We literally hand-walked that drug to approval with a lot of oversight and redundancy." Eyetech got the company running the factory to retain workers by paying them more. Additionally, Eyetech sent its own team to the plant. "We had to get it done. We needed to get approval," Glenn continues, "and the only way we could get it done was through sheer horsepower, through putting our people up there, to this place. It cost us a fortune."

Plugging the brain drain solved a big problem. But another disturbance in Canada shook Eyetech. There was information that the operations in Canada were possibly being sabotaged by a rival. Allegedly, according to a low-level employee in Canada, a competitive company—which, coincidentally, also had a plant in Alberta—fearful of Macugen stealing market share, had apparently paid someone to contaminate Macugen's active pharmaceutical ingredient. An emergency C-suite meeting was convened.

With everyone in the room, the "whistleblower," a guy named Andy,* was put on the phone. After commending Andy's bravery in coming forward,

* Name has been changed for confidentiality and legal reasons.

serious questioning followed. What unfolded, in David's telling, "turned out to be complete garbage. Andy seemed to have made up this whole thing."

If David had any second thoughts about the necessity of finding an alternative manufacturing site, they immediately evaporated. Indeed, looking ahead to meet the anticipated future demand had already led to an acquisition. In late November, Eyetech paid $3 million in cash to Transgenomic for their facility in Boulder, Colorado. Some further investment in infrastructure to produce Macugen at scale was needed, but it was reasonable to expect it would come online shortly after the FDA's pending approval.

Fortunately, the other elements under the purview of CMC quality control went smoothly. Putting the drug into syringes and packaging the works as complete kits with clear labeling was done in California with little fuss. With everything in place for Eyetech, FDA approval became a waiting game.

* * *

For a while, it looked like the clock would run out on 2004 without approval taking place. Then, just before the beginning of the holiday season, the FDA let it be known that their announcement was set to be delivered on Friday, December 17. After a year of getting urgent requests from the FDA for more information about a patient population, or a sub-analysis of one group versus another to understand drug reactions, and endless questions about chemistry, it was down to the wire.

When that day dawned, it was all hands on deck at Eyetech. Surprisingly, the requests kept coming. "We were getting questioned that day and that night up until the last approval minute, which was crazy," explains Loni, who led global regulatory affairs. "You don't expect on the day of approval to get questions." Apparently, someone still had questions about the delivery mechanism, particularly the drug-filled syringe.

Typically, drugs are distributed in vials, and the doctor or whoever is administering the treatment inserts an empty, sterile syringe and then draws up the correct dose before injecting it. With Macugen, a biologically derived substance that has a large molecule, terminal sterilization—where the entire package containing the drug is sterilized, the FDA's preferred method—would cause the protein in the molecule to break down. So, in the case of Macugen, the correct dose was placed in sterile syringes using an aseptic process, meaning it was done in a sterile environment with sterile equipment. But the whole notion of intravitreal injections was new to the FDA.

"I remember everybody sitting in my office the day that we were supposed to get approval," recalls Loni. "And at seven o'clock at night, we still still haven't received the letter." In 2004, the letter was set to come by fax, the noisy machine sitting conveniently behind Loni's desk. Outside, it was dark. Inside, the team was a mixture of nerves and exhaustion, with David still drinking soda while others napped on the floor next to him. Finally, the machine sputtered to life. The entire process from birth to approval was an astoundingly rapid four years, ten months, and eight days. Someone had the good sense to have champagne already chilled. Once again, it was time to celebrate.

Chapter 8

SMOOTH SAILING?

The FDA's approval flipped the switch to "Launch Mode." Anticipating this moment, Eyetech had already hired Paul Chaney as COO to spearhead the initiative. Paul had orchestrated one of the most successful drug debuts in ophthalmology for Xalatan, a glaucoma treatment brought to market by Pharmacia in the 1990s. This achievement earned Paul respect and love across the profession combined with the loyalty of his sales force that was now part of Pfizer. The FDA wasn't entirely in the rear-view mirror, a Phase 2/3 trial for DME was slated for later in 2005, and given the roughly 750,000 active cases of DME in the US alone, David was still keen to pursue that. But as the new year approached, and after such intense pressure to gather, analyze, and present data, with approval for AMD behind them, Eyetech's focus was on successfully getting Macugen into doctors' offices and their patients' eyeballs.

Before champagne corks popped heralding the new year, the December 30, 2004, issue of the *New England Journal of Medicine* featured the Macugen trial results. This prestigious publication, one of the most widely read by doctors around the globe, rolled out the red carpet for the new drug, calling it a "landmark study." The article was careful to dispel any hesitation practitioners may have held concerning intravitreal injections, noting that after administering 7,545 injections, the chance of infection with endophthalmitis was low for patients receiving the drug for a year.

Validation from respected sources is helpful, but nothing beats connecting directly in person. David Hallal, who would go on to be CEO of Alexion and other companies, was brought in to head up sales. Not only did he handpick a great group of reps; he kept them close at hand. David also ensured he would personally meet one-on-one with each of them regularly. The reps loved the singular attention, and David gained great insight to what was happening on the ground. Eyetech's sales force of sixty people fanned out to talk to the two thousand retina specialists in the US, while Pfizer's team, nearly three times the size, tended to general ophthalmologists and the rest of the world. The specialists weren't hard to find. Showing up at the ongoing cycle of ophthalmic scientific meetings and presenting Macugen's case from behind the podium was the surest way to get the word out. Clear science obviated any need for fancy marketing. For a small company with a small sales force, Eyetech managed to punch way above its weight class.

It was also crucial to sell the novel idea of intravitreal injections to a wider audience. Up to this point, only the investigators in the trial had hands-on experience in administering the drug. Part of the presentations involved explaining the intricacies of the drug delivery protocol and introducing doctors to the newly established guidelines. Once again, this task fell to Emmett. "I didn't do it alone," he reflects, "but I spearheaded that. As I look back, I'm quite proud of that." Ultimately, after receiving a small amount of anesthetic by eye drops or a gel, getting a needle in the eye from an ophthalmologist was on par with being injected by a dentist before receiving a filling. This was a manageable level of discomfort everyone could understand.

The global push worked. The proof was in the sales figures. Over the following twelve months, $200 million worth of Macugen was distributed, ranking it as the most successful launch of an ophthalmologic drug ever—a staggering two times the previous record. After decades of being an orphan child in the pharmaceutical world, ophthalmic therapy was finally welcomed into the innermost circle of medicines, ranking in the top 8 percent of all drugs launched in all fields the preceding two decades.

When Eyetech held its first annual general meeting on May 11, it was too early to present the eventual sales figures, but the company's success was evident. Eyetech had the first-mover advantage, valued in financial circles for establishing market share ahead of rivals and building customer loyalty. As the company noted in its annual report, drawing on news reports from around the country, the greatest impact of the drug wasn't just meeting market demand for a blindness treatment but the relief it brought to patients. "I feel that I've certainly been blessed by it and have another chance to have a life because I can read. I could not read before," a patient, Mary Compson, told NBC News. In Florida, the state with the highest percentage of elderly residents, the *Naples Daily News* ran a story titled "Seeing, Believing: New Medications for Macular Degeneration Bringing Hope to Patients." It quoted a patient who said, "It's phenomenal. I can thread a needle. Before Macugen, I could no more have threaded a needle than flown to the moon." Elaborating on the effect of the disease, the patient said, "I couldn't see faces. All colors were hideous; trees and grass were a frosted gray. There was a big round spot in the middle of my vision. It scared me to death." It's easy to count the dollars and cents of Macugen's sales, but quantifying the value of the improved quality of life it brought to sufferers of the disease and their families is beyond measure. The one thing not accounted for at this milestone event was David. He was at a hospital, welcoming his first son, Luca, into the world. Luca was named for Maria's Italian heritage with a middle name Henry, in honor of David's maternal grandfather. Luca was very punctual—being born exactly on his due date. Which just happened to be the same as day as Eyetech's first annual general meeting. A truly priceless moment.

* * *

For David, Tony, and Samir, the success of Macugen was a vindication of their belief that a company led by doctors could thrive in the intensely competitive pharmaceutical business. Their stellar track record on Wall Street also created new opportunities. One way for Eyetech to capitalize on this was to expand its board of directors. As a newly public company, it would be good to have additional members on the board who have experience managing investor relations as well as an extended industry network. The best time to do this was after launching but while they were still on their skyward trajectory.

"So we got a private recruiter to give us names of people who'd be good independent board members," David says of the selection process. "And in general, they identified the sector CEOs of biotech companies, but they also sent other people." Among this latter group of about thirty résumés was a big surprise: Bill Clinton. After the former first couple's move to suburban Chappaqua, north of New York City, and with his wife in the Senate, Bill seemed to be at a loose end. "I guess he was looking for things to do. Why not join some boards?" speculates David. "He was probably thinking more Google than Eyetech. I don't know. But for whatever reason, we were a hot company, and they gave us Clinton's résumé."

You might expect that someone who'd been a governor and president would have a résumé the length of a novel, but for the former leader of the free world, that was not the case. "Here's the thing about it that was really cool," reflects David on his unexpected reading material. "Unlike all these other ten-page résumés, his résumé was one side of one page. It said, 'William Jefferson Clinton,' and for 'operative experience,' it read 'President, United States of America.' Then under that, it said 'military experience: commander in chief, all US military forces.' It was just hysterical how simple it was. Of course, he was much too senior and important for us, but it was nice the recruiter sent it."

A SINGULARITY IN THE MONEY-TIME CONTINUUM

Not long after the annual general meeting, David was back at Scalinatella, the Upper East Side Italian restaurant where he and Marty first discussed Eyetech. David's dining companion this time was Colin Goddard, the CEO of OSI Pharmaceuticals, a New York–based company with a successful lung and pancreatic cancer drug, Tarceva. David knew Goddard from NewYorkBIO, an association for the region's life sciences community. David thought it would be good to have another CEO on the board of Eyetech: "Someone that was pro-management. And who better to know those issues than a CEO?" What David liked about OSI was it had commercialized its drug: "They were a little bit ahead of where we were, that next step up or two." In addition to their companies sharing a similar pharmacological journey, David and Goddard had great personal chemistry.

David had seen to it that other board members felt the same way. Goddard had interviewed with many of them. "Everybody liked him, and they said, 'Yep, we'd love to sign him up,'" remembers David. Taking his fellow CEO to Scalinatella was a warm gesture, the perfect environment to make the offer official. It was bound to be an easy home run. But just as David was winding up his pitch to Goddard, something entirely unexpected happened. Goddard leaned back, picked up his wine glass to take a sip, and said, "Let *me* throw *you* a curve ball. What if instead of joining your board, I bought you?"

David was caught completely off guard. "I was shocked. I didn't see it coming." There was no plan for selling Eyetech. "I had no idea that he was looking to expand his company. This came out of nowhere."

Money is a unique form of energy. It powers the world, surging through finance and trade and driving our economy forward. Day after day. Cash flows. We work. We get paid. We spend. We move along the conveyor belt of consumption. It all feels very linear. However, when money accumulates, it pools, amassing into capital, developing a pecuniary gravity. Banks, institutions, and corporations exert unseen forces, bending the paths of entities passing through the financial system. And just as Einstein said that gravity curves time, at Scalinatella, David discovered that time can be circular, twisted entirely around by money's invisible field. Until this fiscal "singularity," Eyetech had been progressing down the straight path of drug commercialization. Suddenly, the company was ending and beginning anew in the exact same place it started.

David needed some space and time to comprehend what just

happened. It felt like he'd only recently mastered what it was like to raise capital and go through an IPO. (And for a lot of start-ups, their IPO *is* their exit strategy.) In a split second, he needed to become proficient in the art of M&A—mergers and acquisitions. After listening to Goddard's plans, David went home and alerted his board then started lining up bankers. And he made an emergency call to David Redlick. Successfully navigating this new territory was going to require the utmost legal skill, having the best lawyer in biotech on board was essential.

Being drawn into OSI's gravitational pull wasn't the only thing set to radically change Eyetech's trajectory. The ophthalmological firmament was lit up by the birth of a new star. One that would outshine Macugen in unexpected ways.

Lucent [LOO-sent] adj. Glowing. From the Latin *lucere* meaning "to shine"

"This is going to kill Eyetech, unfortunately," Peter Kaiser, a researcher at the Cleveland Clinic and a member of Genentech's scientific advisory board, told *The Wall Street Journal* in a story published on May 24, 2005, just thirteen days after Eyetech's triumphant annual meeting. He was talking about Lucentis, otherwise known as ranibizumab, the Bay Area giant's anti-VEGF AMD treatment. Although Genentech was a long way from presenting Lucentis's Phase 3 results to the FDA, early data from a trial with 716 patients looked very promising. The *Journal* reported that "vision sharpened for at least half the patients getting the drug." The publication also stated, "fully 95% of patients who received Lucentis saw their vision stabilize or improve," comparing this to Macugen's success rate of "just 70% of patients." Nobody needed time and space to gauge the impact of this announcement. As the *Journal* elaborated, Genentech's stock price bounced while Eyetech's fell 30 percent in after-hours trading. The next day it was down by almost half.

In hindsight, Wall Street's immediate response to the news seems completely understandable. But at the time, the science wasn't so clear-cut.

Both drugs were anti-VEGF treatments using the same biological mechanism to treat the same disease. Still, it wasn't entirely evident that analyzing Macugen alongside Lucentis was an apples-to-apples comparison. At the microscopic level proteins work in our bodies, there's a lot of variation. An isoform is a variant of a protein that arises from the same gene but has different genetic coding. Typically, isoforms have distinct lengths and capacities to bind with the anticoagulants in our blood and the supporting structures around our cells. VEGF has four main isoforms: VEGF-A121, VEGF-A165, VEGF-A189, and VEGF-A206. Of these, the most abundant and biologically active is VEGF-A165. This is the one Macugen blocked. "The science suggested there was a safety advantage to blocking only 165; they called it the pathological isoform," explains David. "Lucentis blocked all of them. If you look just at those early preclinical data, you would have said it was better to only block 165. You could get safety problems in the body if you blocked all of it." When Larry Gold at NeXstar built the Macugen molecule, pegaptanib, he was following the science.

"The science doesn't always work," David says equivocally. "Something happened that didn't translate. It's not clear if humans developed compensatory pathways or something that made the other isoforms become more important for efficacy. No one knew definitively. It could have been that the patients were different. You never want to compare patients in different trials." Whatever the reason, David concedes "the data appeared a jump better." People want science to be definitive, to declare an absolute truth, but that's not how it works. When evidence changes, so does science. Science circles the truth, getting closer and closer, zeroing in without ever making contact. Genentech's approach appeared to narrow the gap even further. "What we found in humans, which was a surprise," concludes David, "was that if you blocked all the isoforms, not just 165 like Macugen, you got better efficacy. But would there be a safety advantage to Macugen? That could take years to know."

Lucentis created a lot of noise but didn't interrupt the conversation between Eyetech and OSI. By late August 2005, a deal had taken shape. OSI was offering to buy Eyetech for $20 per share. This was a steep decline from Eyetech's peak at $45 but still a hefty 43 percent premium on its value of $13.99 at closing the day the acquisition was announced and just a dollar below its IPO offering. The deal's total value: $935 million.

Goddard was definitely taking a big risk. Just how big is hard to say. At the time, there was no guarantee Lucentis would be entirely safe. There was some evidence to suggest the drug could harbor possible side effects beyond the concerns of blocking the full array of isoforms. Nasty thromboembolic events like strokes and heart attacks were possible, particularly as wet AMD patients skewed elderly. Of course, when this happens to a patient during a trial, it's extremely hard to determine if it's just random bad luck or the beginning of a pattern. If Lucentis experienced a safety event once it hit the market, there would be plenty of room to compete. Although previously ignored, the market for AMD treatment is huge. In traditional pharmaceutical wisdom, the second-best drug should capture around 20 percent of the market share. Given Macugen's first-mover advantage, some brand loyalty was to be expected, and holding on to a fifth of a billion-dollar market is a nice consolation prize.

Eyetech offered a deeper value, too. OSI began as a one-trick pony, with its drug Tarceva. Then two years before it solicited Eyetech, it created a subsidiary focused on metabolic disorders like diabetes and obesity, but it had yet to bring a drug to market. Operating as an ophthalmic division, Eyetech would add a third leg for even greater stability. "We look at this as the transition of our business beyond the Tarceva success," Dr. Goddard told *The Wall Street Journal*. "We're looking at diversification and scale."

What OSI also faced was competing with its partner—Genentech. In a mirror image of David's experience with interferon, OSI's cancer research was matched with the larger biotech company's ability to conduct clinical trials. Together, the two firms jointly marketed Tarceva in the US, with Roche taking international responsibility. Ironically, erlotinib (the generic name of Tarceva) was developed by OSI with Pfizer. But when

Pfizer merged with Warner-Lambert, in what can be described as a Federal Trade Commission–induced side effect, the junior partner received a royalty-free, cashless license to erlotinib.

Before $935 million can change hands, a lot has to take place. Public companies, like Eyetech, need approval by a majority of shareholders to move forward with a sale. For investors in Eyetech, the 43 percent premium was an attractive off-ramp from a brief but intense roller-coaster ride, Although shareholder approval isn't required to make an acquisition, the story was not so simple for OSI. Despite David and Goddard appearing on CNBC the day the merger was announced, not everyone was as convinced of the deal's virtues as Colin Goddard.

"The deal was controversial from the day we announced it to the day it was completed," reflects Glenn. "Colin was getting beat up all the time by the analysts." As Eyetech's CFO, Glenn was responsible for placing all the financial ducks in a row for the transaction. For Glenn, the joint announcement in late summer led to an entire fall season of negotiations with bankers and lawyers. "It made my career from a deal standpoint because I was the guy with David that negotiated this ironclad deal with OSI."

Today, that deal resides in four giant folders in Glenn's home office, the contents preserved like a chef's collection of favorite recipes. And the pièce de résistance was a series of exceptions to the definition of material adverse changes—MACs in legal parlance, a deal killer in layman's terms. "There were a couple of key MAC exceptions that we negotiated that kind of locked OSI in," he says of his accomplishment.

Despite Eyetech's deft negotiations, dissent from OSI investors wasn't fully quelled. In the period between signing the deal and winning Eyetech's shareholder approval, a warning flashed across the executive team's radar. David recalls, "An investor made a comment, something like, 'If the Raylo manufacturing plant in Canada was destroyed or blown up, would that be a MAC and end the deal?'" The implication that somebody may sabotage and destroy Eyetech's Edmonton operations was clear, albeit seen through a paranoid lens. But with $935 million at stake, paranoia was prudent.

"I then hired a private security company," Glenn says of his rapid response, "a friend of mine who had a big security company, and he goes up and hires Canadian Mounties. Then he got his own people up there." All of a sudden, security became a major line item on Eyetech's budget: "We're spending like $250,000 a month—this obscene amount of money for these armed guards to be there twenty-four-seven walking the perimeter of the building." It was a figure that caught the attention of his counterpart, surveying the outgoings of the company he was acquiring. "I remember the CFO from OSI saying to me, 'Can you tell me what the F these guys with guns are doing walking around the facility?'"

By early November 2005, Eyetech had tabulated its shareholder votes, and its acquisition was resoundingly approved. But OSI was getting cold feet. On November 10, *The Wall Street Journal* ran the headline, "OSI May Be Rethinking Its Merger As Eyetech Drug Faces Competition." According to the *Journal*, this sea change resulted from the November 7 announcement by Genentech "that Phase III clinical trials had shown Lucentis to be highly effective in either improving or maintaining vision in patients with AMD." OSI's board wanted more time to review the Lucentis data. Regardless, Eyetech felt the deal was watertight. This point was reiterated in *The Wall Street Journal* story: "Eyetech believes that it is clear under the merger agreement that OSI has no basis to claim either that a 'material adverse effect' has occurred, or that OSI has any other grounds not to close the merger." This stern warning accompanied Eyetech's acquiescence to give OSI until November 14 but only for its board "to fulfill its fiduciary obligation."

After much nail biting, the deal finally closed on the deadline. Eyetech received $685 million in cash and the balance of the $935 million in OSI's common stock, approximately 5.7 million shares.

MEA CULPA

"Now, it's a shame with Macugen, because it was a great drug. It really was a revolutionary drug," reflects Glenn, almost twenty years after the sale of Eyetech. "Lucentis was just much better."

OSI continued to sell Macugen. In 2006, it netted $107 million from US sales. But that was the end of the line. Almost exactly a year after purchasing Eyetech, on November 6, 2006, OSI decided to divest its eye disease business. Just four months after the June 30, 2006, FDA approval of Lucentis, the show was over.

The evaporating demand for Macugen was highly unusual according to Mike Ross: "If you look at a typical marketed drug that is supplanted in a superiority trial by a slightly better drug, almost all the patients that are on that first drug stay on the first drug. It's not like the drug goes and crashes." However, what Macugen made apparent is that eye doctors are outliers in medicine. "That just doesn't happen in ophthalmology. It's like, 'where's the new shiny penny'? And the rapidity with which Macugen lost market share was dizzying." Looking back at the episode from an investor's point of view, he admits, "Actually, I never would've guessed that was going to happen."

In OSI's annual report for the year, Goddard and the company's chairman, Robert Ingram, detailed what happened in their letter to shareholders. Describing the $935 million Eyetech acquisition as a "misstep" and a "tactical miscue," the letter explains their error: "Our decision to acquire Eyetech was based upon three critical assumptions that have proven to be erroneous." The final false assumption was "that Macugen would have a sustainable niche—based on a preferential safety profile—in the market following the launch of Lucentis." The preceding two assumptions also related to safety. However, not to Lucentis but another Genentech drug, Avastin, one that lacked approval for ophthalmic use. Avastin was a wild card. A wild card on a tear.

Just like interferon, Avastin, an off-label anti-VEGF cancer treatment, was starting to be used by eye doctors. The big difference? Avastin works. Although if one looked at the original science, this wasn't supposed to happen. David explains, "The preclinical science suggested Avastin was likely too big a molecule; it didn't translate to humans. Genentech possibly would've told you, 'Avastin won't work.' They followed the science. And the science was wrong. What people didn't realize, in humans, because of aging, there are likely little rips and tears in the inner limiting membrane—on the surface of the retina between the vitreous and the retina—that nobody thought about. Rips that probably allowed the big antibody Avastin to get in."

This discovery was unorthodox. While Lucentis was on the path to FDA approval, highly respected eye doctors at the Bascom Palmer Eye Institute at the University of Miami took it upon themselves to investigate Avastin's anti-VEGF capabilities. As Philip J. Rosenfeld, MD, PhD, explained in his article published in the May/June 2009 issue of Retina Today, having been involved in the Phase 1 trials for Lucentis, he had approached Genentech in 2003 to see if the company would conduct a clinical trial for intravenous use of bevacizumab (Avastin) for wet AMD. Echoing their response to David four years earlier, the biotech firm answered no.

As Rosenfeld details, in 2004 the FDA issued a warning about bevacizumab. Colon cancer patients had a 1 percent increased risk of thromboembolic events if they were given it biweekly in combination with chemotherapy drugs. Nevertheless, Rosenfeld responsibly persevered, completing a trial with eighteen patients who were made aware of the risk and agreed to treatment. Blood pressure problems were minimal and contained with standard medications. Even though the administration of the drug was systemic, not localized in the eye, the results looked as good as Lucentis.

At the following year's ARVO meeting in Fort Lauderdale in May 2005, Rosenfeld organized a breakfast. Fifty doctors showed up to hear about Avastin's efficacy and safety. But Genentech did not attend. Undeterred, later that month, the doctor gave an intravitreal injection of Avastin to one of his patients, a retired nurse who, despite receiving PDT treatments, was legally blind in one eye and losing sight in the other. As a nurse, she especially understood the risk she was undergoing by taking a drug that had no assurance of safety and gave informed consent. Injecting directly into the eye meant the doctor could use a very small dose, conceivably obviating the concerns about blood pressure. He calculated that even though the Avastin molecule was larger than Lucentis, he would be injecting the same number of molecules in the dosage he devised. The treatment was a success. He tried it on a few more patients with positive results.

Word quickly spread among Rosenfeld's coterie of retinal specialists along with a careful explanation of the injection protocol. By June, this off-label practice was being publicly discussed. In July, more Lucentis data was released, demonstrating that with twelve months of treatment, patients' sight gained an average of 7 letters compared to a loss of 10.5 in the control group. Although Avastin was lacking a large-scale trial, the doctor was able to show that identical processes were occurring with the drug using optical coherence tomography (OCT). The subretinal fluid disappeared, and the macula returned to its normal thickness. News of this success went viral. Ophthalmologists around the world began their own experiments. In a very short time, injecting patients with Avastin morphed from fringe behavior to mainstream practice.

Four years after Avastin's use became widespread, a story covering the ongoing debate about its safety in *EyeNet* magazine asked, "Would the use of Avastin have spread like wildfire if Lucentis, the approved drug for wet AMD, wasn't 40 times more expensive?"

To this day, with numerous FDA-approved treatments for AMD, off-label Avastin still accounts for over 30 percent of the US market.

Doctors shopping for Avastin off-label go to compound pharmacies, specialized pharmacies that create customized medications, usually for patients with unique needs. There they can buy vials of Avastin packaged for oncological use, which are then placed in sterile syringes to give them approximately forty intravitreal doses. "It saves tons of money," says David. "It comes out at something like fifty bucks a shot." When comparing that to the $1900 per 0.5 mg shot for Lucentis, it's easy to see why doctors treating low-income patients and the uninsured in the US opt for Avastin. Similarly, in developing nations, Avastin is the clear winner.

In October 2007, Genentech decided to clamp down on Avastin's off-label use, citing safety concerns. The company halted sales to compound pharmacies. This did not go down well with ophthalmologists or compound pharmacists. At the following month's AAO meeting in New Orleans, a spokesman for the International Academy of Compound Pharmacies declared, "We believe Genentech is putting profit ahead of patients." (Genentech has repeatedly disputed this and any assertion as to its motives in discouraging off-label use is speculative.) A Genentech representative agreed to address the disgruntled eye doctors. The representative showed up with apparent security, as if ready to be confronted by violent ophthalmoscope-wielding assailants. The drug company's heavy-handed optics only exacerbated the enmity. In a rare moment, emotions trumped science, and the doctors apparently heckled the representative. They even booed Napoleone Ferrara at another meeting, winner of the Lasker Award for science, whose research at Genentech straddled both sides of their discontent, the technical foundation supporting both Avastin and Lucentis. Fortunately, cooler heads prevailed, and Genentech ultimately relented and resumed off-label sales.

Eventually, the National Eye Institute studied the effectiveness of Avastin, publishing results in 2012. In this study, it was found to be equivalent to Lucentis. In 2011, Eylea, a drug from Regeneron, was approved for AMD by the FDA, further diluting the marketplace. By the time Eylea arrived, OSI had put Eyetech up for sale. In the end, it was purchased by Valeant Pharmaceuticals from OSI in 2012 for a paltry $22 million, a little more than a fiftieth of its original value.

THE ULTIMATE SATISFACTION

Eyetech's rapid deflation is the inverse of its tremendous impact. Without question, Macugen opened the door for retinal drug development. Lucentis, Eylea, and Vabysmo are FDA-approved wet AMD treatments sharing the market with off-label Avastin today. Would any of these be available without Macugen? Possibly. But how long would we have waited? How many more millions of people would have gone blind? How many grandparents would have never seen their grandchildren's faces? Or not been able to drive them to school? Or help teach them to read?

After Eyetech's acquisition by OSI, David remained as executive vice president for the newly merged entity for six months to help with its transition. He never returned to academia. Instead, Henry Simon, who founded SV Health Investors and was the chairman of Eyetech's board when it was sold, invited David to join SV, the first venture capital firm to invest in Eyetech. Rather than giving lectures to medical students, David found himself being mentored by Henry and Jim Garvey, the firm's managing partner and CEO. Henry's wisdom was very practical, greatly contributing to David's "street MBA." Jim schooled David on his early boards, having gained a wealth of experience in ophthalmic device deals. Over the years, David combined his academic and business skills, resulting in being frequently asked to tell the story of Eyetech, often at investor events, such as giving the keynote at the dinner of MPM Capital's venture fund held during the prestigious JP Morgan Healthcare conference. It's only after attending these types of events that he realized how rare Eyetech's story is—going from birth to IPO in just three years, ten months, and twenty-one days, and then to approval in four years, ten months, and eight days, and finally to being sold in five years, seven months, and twenty days.

Another nine-month journey ended on March 15, 2007. On this momentous day, Maria and David celebrated the birth of their second child, once again a boy. His name was inspired by one of the couple's favorite pursuits—travel. On a vacation in Anguilla, they met a youngster from the UK who seemed to possess something special about him. Their new son also radiated a similar feeling, so they decided to give him the same name, Oliver. And they paired it with the middle name of Matteo, in honor of Maria's Italian heritage—fully expressing their delight in the newborn's initials: OMG!

Joining SV gave David the flexibility to enjoy his expanded family. But it wouldn't be long before David walked through the very door he opened. Except, the next time, he'd be the one carrying the money bag.

Chapter 9

RISK AND REWARD

"It was great," Samir says of the sale of Eyetech and its lasting impact on retinal disease. But success had a counterintuitive effect. "Then it was like, we're all dressed up and nowhere to go. The whole idea was that the shop is closed."

David and Samir weren't so sure. They felt AMD was going to be treated very much like cancer and HIV, where there are multiple targets due to redundancies in the developmental mechanisms of the diseases. Samir summed up their assessment: "There's got to be other assets. Two hits are better than one. Let's just go for it." Only this time, their roles would be reversed. "David was in venture capital, and he said, 'I'll fund you.'"

David was enjoying his new role at SV Life Sciences, the venture capital firm he joined six months after Eyetech's sale. Eyetech running aground in the capital markets in the wake of Lucentis didn't dent David's reputation. "He was a rock star in the venture capital world," Samir confirms. According to him, the investors who got their feet wet early made out like bandits. "I think every VC had their best returns from Eyetech."

Most Monday mornings at seven o'clock, David would fly on the shuttle from New York to Boston, where SV has its headquarters. Meetings started at ten o'clock in the morning to go over the company's entire portfolio with the investment team. Late in the afternoon, he'd return south. Tuesday to Friday he was on his own. Not that David needed any oversight. Never one to be idle, David spent his time working on some of SV's existing investments—both ophthalmological and in other medical areas—plus scouting for opportunities. "You never know how you'll find it," explains David. He stayed alert for any possibilities: "Everything from looking on the internet at a company that has something in their pipeline they may not use, hearing something at a meeting, hearing from a friend, checking your networks at other companies, it's kind of a go for broke."

"What's exciting about it," reflects David, "it's a different play with venture capital. There's always something going on." For David this means everything from being on numerous company boards to receiving enticing emails containing business plans from associates (along with their solicitous calls) and creating start-ups, or NewCos as VCs refer to them. In this case, a VC may build a company, starting with the management team, around an asset. More typically, though, the talent comes first, then comes the search for assets. And this is what David decided to do with Samir. The big difference with funding Samir was that David could also be closer to the ground, something he missed from the usual thirty-thousand-foot view of the VC.

* * *

"I just kept up with the science," Samir recalls, regarding the birth of their next venture. "It was a cloudy day in New York," according to Samir, when David called and told him, "I want you to come up. I have a very good idea." Samir would have preferred to chat on the phone, but David insisted. "No, no, no, we're going to have breakfast."

"I've got all this cash at my disposal to do a new company," David revealed when they met on that chilly day in Manhattan near Columbus Circle. Samir wasn't excited by the prospect. "We just finished Eyetech, and that was one of the most draining experiences," he reminded his friend. Samir was exhausted by the endless yo-yoing of events. He remembered the extreme high of getting a drug approved, which he felt was the absolute acme of wet AMD therapeutics, and its nadir a few weeks later in Montreal when the Lucentis data was revealed, which he felt was, "just like a bomb went off." This was all capped by what Samir called "the most magical sale ever done in history that Eyetech pulled off with

OSI." They still needed to recover from the Eyetech journey. "It took a lot out of me," he reflects, "took a lot out of David and Tony, everybody. It was just really brutal."

Samir likened the notion of starting another company to running a four-hundred-meter dash immediately after completing a marathon. "Just the thought of it," he remembers, "I felt like running away." In the end, Samir told his friend as they left the restaurant, "I've got to think about it." David, true to character, was unrelenting, replying, "There's nothing to think about." He persisted, repeatedly striking Samir on the shoulders of his down parka with both hands like an antagonistic coach giving a pep talk. "Yeah, you can do it; we can do it. We'll put a team together. This is very, very easy." Samir was unconvinced. As usual, rather than taking no for an answer, David simply diluted his request to make it easier to swallow. Finally, he proposed, "Just look for assets. Okay? We'll do the rest afterwards."

For the next nine months, the pair of ophthalmologists scoured the world, investigating hundreds of possible chemicals for likely therapeutics. At the conclusion of this exhaustive search, they realized the answer had been right in front of them the whole time, developed by Tony and his team at Eyetech. It was an anti-PDGF (platelet-derived growth factor) drug, Fovista or pegpleranib. The purpose of the drug was to strip pericytes, isolated cells on the walls of capillaries, and allow for a more potent anti-VEGF attack. It would be part of a combination therapy, adding a different action to make anti-VEGF drugs work even better. OSI bought it along with the rest of Eyetech. But OSI's rapid exit from ophthalmology meant the company was happy to surrender it back to David and Samir, for little more than a royalty once sales hit a certain level.

With an asset in hand, David felt it was time for his venture company to front some seed money. There was a meeting with SV, and funding was okayed. This time the investment would be led by Lutz Giebel, who received his PhD in molecular biology at the University of Heidelberg then studied human genetics at the University of Wisconsin in Madison before joining

SV to focus on bio-therapeutics. "Lutz was great to work with," recounts David, "very logical and practical." The meeting concluded with an understanding that the nascent team would secure a second asset in short order. Samir maintained this next asset should be a complement inhibitor.

The complement system is part of the body's immune system. Composed of a group of proteins, it works to fight infection and remove damaged cells. In April 2005, Samir had seen an issue of *Science* magazine with three independent studies showing that polymorphisms in the gene coating for a complement were associated with both wet and dry AMD. When he looked deeper into the research, Samir concluded that complement-mediated inflammation was responsible for the onset of AMD. Stop the inflammation and you'll stop AMD, he theorized. David would always say, "No one is better at finding assets than Samir."

There was a company, Alexion, who was already venturing down this path. A study they did with a complement inhibitor in association with the University of Miami achieved negative results. But Samir wasn't discouraged by this. The doses were given intravenously (systemically), but, he reasoned, given Eyetech's experience, the drug would only work if injected directly into the eye. Alexion's molecule, a full antibody, was a large one; a smaller molecule might also be more conducive. David and Samir decided to approach Archemix, a Cambridge, Massachusetts–based company specializing in producing aptamers that had Mike Ross on its board. They had already sourced Archemix to create the anti-PDGF aptamer, so it seemed like a natural fit. This new aptamer from Archemix would target the C5 protein in the complement system, a protein crucial to responding to infection and inflammation.

What was scarcely more than a dream, with two assets in possession, now became a reality. All it needed to manifest itself was a name. As the sale to OSI proved, having *tech* as a suffix had outlived the stigma of the dot-com crash. Leaning toward science more than poetry, the company became Ophthotech.

BLAST OFF

"Ophthotech was like a rocket ship," says David. "Samir got tremendous funding from the top VCs." At any other time, this might not have been as extraordinary. While the dot-com crash had long faded from view by early 2007, there were rumbles in the financial system, foretelling the advent of a much larger economic earthquake.

Beginning in late 2006, people with lower incomes began to default on their mortgages. Often saddled with inferior credit ratings, these new borrowers had been enticed into the early-2000s frothy real estate market with variable interest rates and reduced collateral requirements. Lenders, on the other hand, were seduced by the proliferation of mortgage-backed securities (MBS), which bundled mortgages of various qualities together and divided them into tidy institutionalized investment vehicles, ostensibly spreading risk while providing attractive returns. The MBS business was brisk. Following the repeal of the Glass-Steagall Act in 1999, there was little separating investment banking from commercial banking; the hard-won wisdom brought forth in the aftermath of the crash of 1929 was deemed senile seventy years later. And now, unconstrained, Wall Street was having a field day. Until the first harbinger of a bust occurred on March 8, 2007. On that day, New Century Financial, the country's leading independent originator of subprime mortgages, stopped accepting loan applications. Ninety-six hours later, the New York Stock Exchange ceased trading its shares following an 89 percent decline in price. On April 2, New Century filed for bankruptcy. The contagion spread quickly through the financial world. By mid-July, Bear Sterns, the fifth largest investment bank, revealed its two subprime hedge funds had lost almost their entire value. The stage was set for the biggest system collapse since the Great Depression.

Against this darkening financial backdrop, the money allowed Samir to do some small trials with around twenty patients. He conducted the first intravitreal injection of a complement inhibitor for dry AMD. "I had to try to get as much efficacy as I could," Samir says of the limited trial. "And we saw what David terms as an on/off effect, meaning you give the drug for three doses and then stop. The growth was paralleling. The decrease of growth was when we gave the medication, and when we ceased, the growth took off. There was definitely a signal." Clearly, there was some potential, but it was the other drug, the anti-PDGF treatment soon to be known as Fovista, that really caught their attention. "The Fovista first trial," David put simply, "looked really good." It was something powerful to attract key investors. At least any who had managed to hold on to their money.

"The promising Phase 1/2 data was interesting because that was the year when American finance was upside down," Samir recalls. "In 2007 nobody could raise one cent of capital, let alone banks were going out of business. But I did the only pari-passu round, and we had eight term sheets." (*Pari passu*, Latin for "equal footing," means all investors are treated equally.) From across the spectrum of doctors, consultants, and venture capitalists, the response was universal: "Everybody thought Fovista was great."

Around $30 million was needed to get things moving. SV took the lead, but a syndicate was necessary to achieve this target. "David had the contacts," relates Samir, "because he was already in venture capital. He says, 'Samir, you've got to meet this guy and pitch him a story; here's his contact number.'" Although Samir had never heard of this European-based investment group before, he placed the call. Then he heard a familiar word: *airport*. Once again, it was the signal for immediate action. But this time, it was Samir's turn to rush. He needed to pitch the guy before he boarded a flight to Copenhagen.

"I went to Newark Airport," Samir says of his escapade to Delta Air Lines' hub in Terminal 2. "He'd already checked in; he was going through security when I stopped him, and just before the security entrance, I'm presenting him a slide deck on our new assets and what the company is going to look like and why we are the best people." This was enough to secure the unfamiliar gentleman's interest and put the TSA on hold. The potential investor, Thomas Dyrberg of Novo Ventures, the venture arm of the Danish financial firm Novo Holdings, agreed to sit down and chat. At a semicircular burger joint near the entrance to the security area, the two men reached a tentative deal. "It was wild," reflects Samir. For the CEO of a company yet to establish an office, he was off to a flying start.

Another key investor was Clarus, a life sciences investment firm run by Nick Galakatos. (Clarus was acquired by Blackstone in 2018 to launch its life sciences group.) Not only did Galakatos contribute financially; he also took Samir under his wing. "Nick was very instrumental in being a mentor to me and eventually a friend," says Samir about their relationship. "He was very hands-on with a tremendous amount of experience and a lot of excellent ideas." HBM Partners also joined the syndicate.

GETTING THE BAND BACK TOGETHER

From his perch as chairman of the board, David viewed the birth of this new company with avuncular pride. Selling Eyetech was emotional as much as financial for him. "You kind of feel like you lost your baby," he reflects. "There's something really nice about having a company." Being on the venture capital side was enjoyable, but it wasn't the same. "You want to have it again," he remembers. Ophthotech was the best of both worlds. David once again had two jobs—one in VC and a very active daily role as chairman: "Even though I wasn't CEO, as the chairman and with Samir doing it and bringing back a lot of the same people, it was almost like, 'You did bring it back.'"

Evelyn wasn't so sentimental about the good old days of Eyetech, even if it was tons of fun. "Oh, I'm happy to say that I went into retirement," she says in reference to her career move after Eyetech. Her stock options in Eyetech created what she called "life-changing money." But she harbored a suspicion her new station among the leisure class was bound to be brief. "David had made me promise him that before I took another job, I would call him." Sure enough, retirement was short-lived. "I never got to the point of calling him. Because he called me."

"He said to me, 'Okay, you've been off nine months or ten months,'" recounts Evelyn of David's invocation. "You're too young to retire. You need something to do. I have this opportunity for you: the COO of Ophthotech, this new company." Having grown accustomed to the pleasure of her own thoughts, she needed a moment to wrap her head around his proposition. "And I said, 'Well, I've never been a COO before. There's a lot of things that I don't know. I don't know the business, the BD part. I don't know the manufacturing part. I don't know the QA part.'" But she was clear about her areas of expertise: "I know the drug development, the clinical operations, and development part. I know that area. I wanted to be very upfront and honest and transparent." David took Evelyn's hesitation in stride. "Don't worry about it," he reassured her. "We'll teach you that part. We'll educate you; you'll learn that part." David thought about his medical training, where the expression summarizing learning was "See one, do one, teach one." Passing on the knowledge he'd gained from Marty and John was the same. Listening between the lines, Evelyn discerned what David was after. "I think," she explains, "what he felt is that they really needed someone who had the people skills to bring on a team and lead the team, especially early on." Besides, the title on offer didn't sound so bad, either. "So I took that job as the COO."

Immediately, things shifted into high gear. Loni da Silva returned as SVP of global regulatory affairs, joined by other pharma industry veterans, including Keith Westby for project management, and Doug Kornbrust, an expert in preclinical toxicology. "We started out with a very small office at One Penn Plaza on the thirty-fifth floor," explains Evelyn. "And then Samir acquired space in Princeton. Because Samir lived in Princeton, and he wasn't going to commute every day." Quickly, roles became established for the two locations. In Princeton, data management, regulatory affairs, QA, and manufacturing congregated around Samir; the clinical operations, development, and safety folks made their headquarters in Manhattan. Just like at Eyetech, workspace rapidly evaporated as more staff came on board. Evelyn remembers during the build-up over the various trial phases moving three times in the same building. “We had walls knocked down; we continued to build and build and build.”

The impetus behind this activity was the largest Phase 2b trial to be conducted in retina to date. The trial’s goal was to show that using Fovista in combination with Lucentis, or similar anti-VEGF treatments, would prohibit subretinal fibrosis, the formation of scar tissue beneath the retina and potentially address anti-VEGF resistance (when some eyes are not as responsive to anti-VEGF monotherapy). Collectively this could result in enhanced vision. When subretinal fibrosis happens in patients, it’s a key predictor of a poor outcome despite treatment with anti-VEGF therapies. Arresting the development of subretinal fibrosis would be a huge improvement for a large number of AMD sufferers. Indeed, if the Phase 1 trial results could be replicated—showing unprecedented visual gain accompanied for the first time by robust neovascular regression, that is, the shrinking of diseased blood vessels—this combination therapy had the potential to become the standard of care. In other words, it could piggyback on Lucentis all the way to the bank.

This possibility had investors salivating. But along with heightened expectations comes pressure. With Eyetech’s success in the rearview mirror and the prospect of achieving an equal or even more spectacular outcome stretching before him, Samir was driven to perform at the highest level. “It was very typical,” Samir says of his CEO workload. “I would literally put in ninety hours a week.” His style was to get involved in every aspect of running the business: “Even the presentations, I did all of the regulatory agencies outside the US.” Samir was intimately familiar with all the details, from the preclinical to the statistical. He would walk into a conference room with a table surrounded by chairs, the expectation that the information about to be received would be delivered by a large team; however, with Samir at the helm, many of the chairs remained empty.

Samir created the company logo. For him, this was a manifestation of true entrepreneurial spirit: “We did everything in-house. I mean, both drugs were named by my wife. Every press release—we wrote it. It was all done by ourselves." Once he received an email from the head of the Committee for Medicinal Products for Human Use the European Medicines Agency's committee responsible for drugs, inquiring about his personal health, asking him, "Do you ever sleep?"

According to Evelyn, the answer was often no. "He wouldn't sleep sometimes for forty-eight hours. He wouldn't sleep." This unrelenting focus was also asked of the people Samir led. "He expected everybody else to work like that," reflects Evelyn on the company culture. "When the company formed, his slogan was: We're 24/7. We're 24/7." The result was a constant sense of urgency. At any time, something important may require immediate attention. "You would get an email from Samir," recounts Evelyn, "and it would say, *please call*." The pressure was constant. Sometimes this meant being contacted while vacationing, celebrating a milestone birthday on a catamaran in the Caribbean, or while hiking in the mountains, prompting a nervous scurry in search of sufficient cell phone service to join a meeting.

CAPITALIZING ON IMMINENT SUCCESS!

Despite the intense pressure and unlike Macugen's breakneck speed, Fovista's development moved along at the customarily slow pace of modern pharmaceuticals. Conducting a traditional, controlled, Phase 2b trial with 449 patients in 69 centers in North America, South America, Europe, and Israel—the largest ever for AMD—was a painstaking process. But the data showed it was exceptionally positive. Even before the fanfare of the official announcement, word started to circulate.

As the ARVO meeting in Fort Lauderdale in May 2012 loomed, Ophthotech prepared to issue a press release on Monday the seventh, the second day of the gathering. "As a courtesy to the FDA," recounts David, "we wanted to tell Wiley Chambers, the FDA ophthalmics head, before it became public. So, we contacted him on the Friday and said, 'Hey, we'd like to take some time to tell you about the data over the weekend if you're at ARVO.'" David and Samir expected a cursory response from him suggesting a quick encounter in a hallway between events. "Instead," says David, "Wiley goes, 'I'm flying up Saturday night. I land about eight o'clock. What if I come straight from the airport to your hotel?'" It sounded extraordinary. "And we were blown away."

Now, the tables were turned. Samir and David were worried. How would this appear to people? "Where are we going to meet him?" They wondered. "We can't meet him downstairs." The best place to avoid unwanted attention was in their hotel room. But that also seemed weird—the head of the FDA Ophthalmics coming to their room. Still, what choice did they have?

Later, they anxiously waited in Samir's room for a tap on the door. "David had consumed seven Diet Cokes by then and was as hyper as you can get," Samir remembers. "And sure enough, the door knocks, and here he comes. We're petrified." It showed the tremendous dedication of Wiley Chambers, who was willing to get off a plane and immediately go look at the data. Of course, it was actually an informal doctor-to-doctor meeting more than a regulatory interaction.

They showed Wiley Chambers what they had: some very detailed slides with imagery and statistics. After twenty-four weeks, compared to AMD patients receiving only standard anti-VEGF treatment, the ones who received Fovista in addition to anti-VEGF therapy were just half as likely to experience progression of their subretinal fibrosis. In other words, doubling up with Fovista on top of Lucentis was twice as good. And for patients who didn't yet have any scarring under their retina, it was five times less likely that they develop fibrosis when using both drugs rather than solely using Lucentis. All in all, the study concluded that the combined drugs provided a 62 percent relative visual benefit over anti-VEGF monotherapy. Safety is, of course, always a major concern to the FDA, but no significant issues were observed for either treatment group in the trial. Samir and David knew the data was good, but they still weren't ready for Dr. Chamber's response. It came as a question: "Why did you stop here?"

The man who the American Academy of Ophthalmologists described as "a guiding force" during the expansion of "our ophthalmologic treatment arsenal" continued to explain his reasoning, telling David and Samir, if they had gone three more months, it may have counted as one of the two pivotal Phase 3 trials.

"We looked at each other, just completely stunned," Samir says of his and David's reaction. Just three more months and Fovista might have been halfway through Phase 3. "It was truly amazing. At that point, we just felt like we walked on water." This was as close as you could get to a great endpoint with a Phase 2 trial.

Granted, this was a highly informal review, under very unusual circumstances that carried no legitimate weight, but it was a tremendous vote of confidence for David and Samir. Enough for the pair to change their strategy. One of the most significant things that was very different in 2012 from the beginning of Ophthotech five years earlier was the state of the economy. With data this good, they could adopt a more vigorous approach to fundraising. The sooner Fovista was in Phase 3, the better!

The first step was to go back to their original investors and see if they could up their ante. Novo was in. Before the end of the month, the Danes had agreed to an additional $125 million in exchange for royalties of Fovista sales, topped off with another $50 million in the form of Series C preferred stock. At the same time, Ophthotech's board decided they should put their best financial foot forward by installing David, with his financial experience, as CEO while leaving Samir as president, allowing him to focus fully on clinical development, his area of expertise. Samir was also given the role of vice chairman of the board.

Samir sees the change of leadership as reflecting a different path the company would now take: "The idea when we started Ophthotech was never to go it alone. It was to get the proof of concept at Phase 1 and then do an M&A." Having such strong data presented the possibility of going public, just like Eyetech. David, as the face of the company, would be instantly familiar to Wall Street. But at the end of the day, it was their combined efforts that counted. "Having two individuals with complementary skill sets is the greatest thing," Samir summarizes. They may have swapped positions, but it was still teamwork that would win the day. "It was a complete co-leadership," emphasizes David. "Samir really being the genius. And my job in that stage was really just making sure the operations and everything went smoothly." They felt they exemplified the notion of great minds thinking alike. "Samir and I were always in sync. We both came to the same conclusions before one of us could even finish asking the question on any topic."

A sure sign that wooing Wall Street was now top priority was inviting Glenn Sblendorio to join Ophthotech's board in 2013. While still serving as president of the Medicines Company—garnering experience that would come in very handy in the not-too-distant future at Ophthotech—Glenn was put in charge of the transaction committee, helping to tee up the coming IPO playing a supporting role to David and Samir. The roadshow to investors was a repeat performance of Eyetech: intense, hectic, and punctuated with delicious food. There were insanely tasty pretzels in Germany, mountains of premium cheese in London, deep-dish pizza in Chicago (of course), and David's favorite Mexican cuisine in San Francisco. Along the way, David ensured that his team—and himself in particular—was fueled by a bottomless supply of Coke Zero, which he personally escorted through airport security in bulk and onto the private jets speeding them to the next meeting. But the real star of the show was the data. "We gave more data out than anyone. It was a very, very packed data set," Samir says of their presentations. Although they had done the rounds of the ophthalmological conference circuit with gusto, Samir remembers the intensity of the roadshow: "We presented it everywhere. There was never more of a display than the roadshow."

The data drove investment. By the middle of August, Ophthotech was ready to file for its initial public offering, with Morgan Stanley and JP Morgan jointly bookrunning. Toward the end of the next month, the price for 8.74 million shares of common stock was set at twenty-two dollars per share, a dollar more than Eyetech's price almost a decade ago. In a sequel to Eyetech, the whole crew were back at the NASDAQ building in Times Square for the big day on September 25. David with Samir at his side, surrounded by their company, rang the opening bell, setting off a flurry of confetti. Oversubscribed by a multiple of twenty-four, action on the exchange was vigorous. At the close of trading, Ophthotech had raised $192 million, achieving a market capitalization of $622 million. "You just never get an IPO like that, where you get that kind of oversubscription and that kind of a hit rate. Like one in a billion," muses David about the market euphoria. "Being able to do that twice was pretty crazy."

* * *

Ophthotech was now extraordinarily well funded going into its Phase 3 trials for Fovista. In keeping with this robust backing, the company planned to cover all contingencies by conducting a trio of investigations with 1,866 patients spread across 225 centers around the globe. In an effort to ensure the combination therapy was agnostic to the type of anti-VEGF treatment patients received, the first two trials focused on combining Fovista with Lucentis and the third trial was Fovista used with either Eylea, Regeneron's anti-VEGF drug approved in late 2011, or Avastin, the unapproved but profoundly popular off-label Genentech upstart, which had gobbled up 60 percent of the market. The goal was to have all the trials' topline data gathered and analyzed by 2016.

Confidence in Ophthotech's triple-pronged approach was so strong that the biotech start-up possessed an almost magnetic appeal. As patients signed up for the Phase 3 trials, one of the world's top drug companies made an irresistible overture. In May 2014, Switzerland-based Novartis sought to enhance Fovista's anti-VEGF agnosticism, potentially giving physicians an even greater choice by offering them a co-formulation. The idea being to provide Fovista together with an anti-VEGF made by Novartis readily mixed in a prefilled syringe. This would be marketed as an alternative to one just containing Fovista, which Novartis would also manufacture and distribute outside of the US. The terms of this ex-US deal were particularly sweet: $200 million upfront, plus another $130 million in enrollment-based milestone payments during the Phase 3 trial. Plus, it meant that Ophthotech would retain everything in the US. And that's not all. For reaching marketing targets outside the US, there would be payments totaling as much as $300 million; additionally, ex-US sales could bring another $400 million—and then they were royalties, too. All up, it was a billion-dollar-plus deal—potentially. "It showed a lot of excitement for the drug," reflects David, modestly. "I have to say, it's a lot of money. And it showed validation of the science by Novartis." David attests, "Bruce Peacock did an amazing job negotiating this deal."

* * *

In the company's Midtown office at One Penn Plaza, an alternative approach to funding had been organized. This wasn't a top-down effort from senior management but a grassroots collective. A group of office workers pooled their resources to play lotto—they called themselves the "Lucky 16 Trust." Every week for five years, they diligently followed a protocol: Members would chip in four dollars and then, in their unique way, randomize the ticket-buying process by going to a different store. On Tuesday, March 24, 2015, two levels below and around the corner from Ophthotech's office, a lotto ticket was acquired from Carlton Cards. The following Thursday, the numbers 02–23–32–45–55 and Mega Ball 12 were drawn.

"There was a lot of buzz around the office following the drawing as everyone learned the jackpot winner was sold in our building," Evelyn told *The New York Post*. "A few of us decided we should probably check our numbers." They did. A few times. Going from computer to computer. Nobody could believe their luck. The $58 million Mega Millions jackpot was theirs. After taxes, each of the sixteen received a more-than-tidy $1.65 million. They called a meeting in their conference room, but they didn't sit around discussing much—they just jumped for joy!

Getting a drug from the lab to approval has about a one in ten chance. Winning the Mega Millions lotto has something along the lines of a one in 300 million chance. Even if you do it every week for five years, you don't move the probability needle. Suddenly having $1.65 million extra is a life-changing event. For the management of Ophthotech, there now was a new risk: that a large number of employees would decide that altering the trajectory of their own lives by retiring on the spot was more important than launching a life-changing drug to treat other people's blindness. Fortunately, for David and Samir, this wasn't the case. The lucky sixteen all stayed on. Why not strive for more than one life-changing event?

While Ophthotech's employees dealt with their own unanticipated bonanza, senior management realized the company's anticipated bonanza had to be carefully managed. Before the Phase 3 trials were completed, Ophthotech lured Glenn away from his position as president and CFO at the Medicines Company to become executive vice president and chief operating officer. "My objective at Ophthotech when I joined in April of 2016 was to help the company commercialize," says Glenn of his move. He was focused on planning the manufacturing and on stewarding the complex relationship with Novartis. Everything had to be in place before the Phase 3 data was released in the final quarter of the year.

THIS CAN'T BE REAL

Call it a ritual, a ceremony, a rite, or whatever term thoroughly scientific people use to describe the routines they perform to ensure good luck; that's what David and Samir did on Friday, December 9, 2016, the day the Phase 3 results for the two trials of Fovista with Lucentis were set to come out. Like during previous data releases, they met at David's apartment, dressed in the same Eyetech-logo clothes they always wore for such auspicious revelations. As they walked to David's home office, the hallowed ground where they would receive the biostatistician's wisdom, David's wife, Maria, presented them with a book, inscribed "Dave and Sam Do it Again."

With so much riding on the outcome, the last thing David and Samir wanted was to be swamped with statistical minutiae. Like always under these circumstances, the statistician was to present them the probability value, or P value—the measure of success—first, on its own. Equal to or less than 0.05 and the trial was a success. Meaning there was a 5 percent or lower probability that the observed effect was due to chance. The FDA's cut-off point. More than 0.05 and the trial failed to demonstrate a statistically significant benefit. The P value would be on the top right corner of the very first slide in the presentation deck. Success was simple to see. A positive result—the trial achieved statistical significance—was displayed as an asterisk. The two doctors were ready, focused on the top right corner of the screen. Just signal. No noise. "Click on it," Samir says of the reductive simplicity.

In front of the computer screen in David's library, Samir had a momentary flash of nerves: "I had brought in so many investors. I was like, my God, I have to face these people if it's negative."

David remained confident: "Everyone in the world thought our drug, Fovista, was going to work."

Click.

The asterisk was NOT there!

For the first trial, the P value was 0.44. Put simply, a 44 percent chance the result was achieved by luck alone. In other words, the trial failed to prove the combined drugs were more effective than simply using Lucentis alone.

"It was just unbelievable," recalls Samir. "The first thing I thought, there's a typo. The statistician just didn't understand what he was doing, what our instructions were."

Then the same thing happened with the second trial, only worse. Its P value was 0.71.

None of the results bore any statistical significance. It was unequivocal. Fovista didn't work. There was no difference between the control group and the treatment group.

The next thing Samir did was call Wiley Chambers. Even though it was a Friday evening, the FDA director answered. “Wiley?” Samir asked frantically, “How can this be possible with the amazing Phase 2b results we had in the last trial? This is just impossible. Have you ever seen anything like it?”

It took Dr. Chambers a moment to reply; he thought he could recall, maybe one time.

Looking back on this dramatic occasion years later, Samir still feels the weight of disappointment: “It was just a heartbreak. Really a heartbreak.”

David likens his emotional reaction to Tom Brady losing the Super Bowl. “You’re like a quarterback who’s confident of winning. Then for days and weeks, you cannot believe you actually lost. You feel stunned.” Fleshing out his thoughts, David continues, “No one does a Phase 3 trial if they are not pretty confident that their drug works—that is, no one thinks they have an ugly baby.”

DICE, COINS, CARDS, AND DRUGS

If humans truly understood probability, there would be no casinos, and Wall Street would resemble Washington, DC, or more likely Arlington, Virginia, or perhaps, Bethesda, Maryland—the preferred domiciles of the nation’s top bureaucrats, the antithesis of financial risk-takers. It’s no secret that modern culture celebrates dice rollers more than pencil pushers. The reason capitalism rewards risk is because of the possible downside: the greater the chance of failure, the higher the reward for success. Which is just magnificent when you’re successful. But no matter how data driven we become, success and desire will always be intimately connected. We all know desire is anything but rational.

“We ran the trials and everybody was like, ‘Was it going to be unbelievable, or was it going to be just very good?’” says David about the enthusiasm for Fovista. “And then when it failed, everyone was shocked.”

Comparing the Macugen experience with Fovista reveals a paradox for David: "At Eyetech, we were rookies from academia. We really didn't know a lot about drug development. We did thirty patients, no controls. We went straight to Phase 3—something rarely done—and we won! The second time around with some drug development experience behind us, we actually went the other extreme. We did the most conservative trial ever. The largest Phase 2b ever done. Four-hundred-plus patients, controls, it worked. And then the drug failed in Phase 3. You would've expected the opposite." David notes, "Any Phase 3 is fifty-fifty, like tossing a coin." But given the very positive results of Phase 2b for Fovista, David had different expectations: "You've got to think it's much higher, certainly a lot better chance to win than the thirty uncontrolled patients from Macugen. It's ironic."

Drug development as a whole is a very risky business. At the first stage, only a tiny percentage of drugs make it out of the laboratory and into clinical trials. A study in biostatistics from the Oxford University Press in 2018 analyzed approval success rates as drugs progressed through the trial process. Drugs for different diseases vary in their journeys, and there are multiple pathways to follow. However, after analyzing the trial data for 21,143 compounds across fifteen years, the researchers drew some general conclusions. In Phase 1, the odds of getting to Phase 2 vary tremendously, as essentially researchers are mostly looking for an indication of its effect. Generally, Phase 2, which weeds out drugs for lack of efficacy or potent side effects, is typically the toughest, with around a 30 percent chance of success. Phase 3 is a little more forgiving; close to 50 percent of drugs make it through. Just as in David's coin toss analogy.

But if you look at the possibility of success from the outset, the overall chances aren't great. If a drug makes it out of the lab, it ultimately has only a 10 percent chance of reaching approval. Think of all the money and time lost on those other nine drugs that don't get there. That's a very real risk known to everyone in biotech. It's little wonder that after all the expense it takes to get a drug approved, when approval happens, it feels like hitting the jackpot.

For David and Samir, the failure of Fovista's Phase 3 trials felt catastrophic. In reality, they simply called heads and got tails.

THE AFTERMATH

When a billion dollars is riding on a coin toss and you lose, don't expect empathy from your backers. (Depending on what factors are included, the average cost of developing a drug from the laboratory to approval ranges from $870 million to $1.8 billion.) "At the end of 2016, the investor reaction was visceral," remembers Glenn. "It's angry. Really, really bad. Of course, the stock takes a huge downturn."

There was one last glimmer of hope, the final trial combining Fovista with Eylea or Avastin. When its results came out in August 2017, it, too, was a dud. Headlines like "Ophthotech Completes Clean Sweep of Phase 3 Trial Flops" in biotech industry publications didn't help, but that was just rubbing salt into the wound. The damage was already done.

Samir felt badly bruised by the disappointment. He had so much riding on the result. In France, independent verification of the outstanding Phase 2b data led to him being honored as "le Parrain de la Maculaire" or "the Godfather of Macula." But the Phase 3 results left Samir feeling like Don Vito Corleone after getting nearly assassinated on a New York street.

The scary thing is how closely real life came to resemble fiction. Samir received threatening phone calls. Given the dire financial circumstances, the company decided to take the threats seriously and hired bodyguards for both Samir and David. For David, the experience was surreal: "I was going home in the subway, and they wouldn't let me leave until there was a bodyguard who went in the subway with me." Even though his defender was heavily built, David found the whole thing perplexing. "He was dressed undercover. If I had to guess who was the bodyguard in the subway, I'd never imagine it was him. And he wasn't standing right next to me. It was just kind of so weird. I'm on the subway; this is crazy."

A few days later, David went on a ski trip in Utah with his family.

"We're going to get you bodyguards there until we know what this is about," David was told. Despite his own skepticism and his wife's incredulity, they had a guard stationed outside their condo. "24/7, there's someone in the hallway by our door," remembers David. "How do I explain this to my kids?" Even more surprising to David was the bodyguard's inquiry when they checked in: "Can I speak with you for a minute?" the guard asked him. David momentarily stepped away from his family. David continues, "And the bodyguard looks at me and says, 'I just need to know, are you armed?'" It took David aback: "And I'm like, 'Am I armed? I've never touched a gun in my life!'" A few days into the trip, with no threat materializing, David felt the whole situation was absurd and asked for his protection to be dismissed. The whole scenario seemed like an overreaction.

At some point, David recalls a private detective was brought in and eventually the perpetrator was uncovered: a very disgruntled retail investor. Apparently, he was intimidated enough by being identified and was never heard from again.

* * *

Fortunately, the threats never led to any physical action. But emotionally wounded, Samir decided to depart from Ophthotech's management team before 2017 to spend time with his father who was getting sick and tend to other important family needs.

Evelyn, too, was crushed by the negative results. "I had never really experienced that low; a low like that," she says, reliving the pain. "I'm telling you; I was depressed." During all her time in the industry, she had been fortunate to avoid failures: "There was one drug I worked on; it failed for one indication—a bone marrow transplant—but it was approved for another indication. It worked for solid organ transplant." Fovista's failure cut to her core: "That hit me like a ton of bricks."

Ophthotech as a company started to crumble, and Evelyn was saddled with taking apart the pieces she was responsible for. "I had to lay off a whole lot of people," she says, conjuring up the unpleasant memory. From a team of about 160 people, all that remained she describes as "a skeleton crew, certain people that hung in there."

The company was built on more than one asset. But with all the attention on Fovista, the C5 complement inhibitor, which at that time was called Zimura, was treated like an orphan child. "We kind of finished off the C5 program," Evelyn notes of the lack of interest. "It was 'tick the box' to finish the early stages." At the board level, David felt isolated. "I was by myself. Nobody else on the board appeared to really want to study Zimura like I did," he reflects on his predicament. "I was likely perceived as a pain at the board meeting. They apparently just finally said, 'Fine, we'll just do this little trial.'"

Could Ophthotech be salvaged? All the deals built on Fovista were null and void. The Danish medical trade press ran headlines like "Ophthotech failure cancels out Novo Ventures' biggest investment," describing the firm's $125 million outlay as "rendered virtually worthless." Ophthotech's stock was in the toilet. The company had laid off a large portion of its staff, down to a core of about twenty people, but despite all that, it was sitting on a pile of cash, around $200 million.

Chapter 10

NOT A ONE-TRICK PONY

Changes were made at Ophthotech. On January 1, 2017, Glenn would take over from Samir as president while continuing as COO, and wanted to change the company's direction. He wanted to pivot to gene therapy. Glenn felt this burgeoning area of research held great promise. Gene therapy, he believed, would prove the source for new approaches in eye care. The FDA was on track to approve the first gene therapy–based drug, Kymriah, developed by Novartis for a specific type of leukemia in August 2017, and Luxturna, a treatment for a rare inherited form of blindness, would get the FDA's nod by the end of the year. Although gaining increasing attention, the gene therapy field was still wide open in Glenn's assessment. Other than Spark Therapeutics, the makers of Luxturna, there was no viable competition yet. A cashed-up Ophthotech could make real headway.

David remained somewhat skeptical. He felt gene therapy was mostly going to address small "orphan diseases," ones that affected fewer than two hundred thousand people in the US, nothing like the market for AMD and DME. But following Fovista, David's opinion apparently now carried less weight in the boardroom. Still, as CEO, he insisted on continuing to move ahead with the complement inhibitor. Why throw away good science? In what David considered a gesture of appeasement, an agreement was made that the development of Zimura would go on in the background, with the focus on gene therapy. No one ever imagined what that little appeasement would ultimately be worth.

As 2017 progressed, Glenn's business development team was busy discovering and sifting through the gene therapy targets while Evelyn's team prepared for the next Zimura trial. For a long time, Zimura's development had been a slow burn, but even with the focus on gene therapy, the team brought in Tom Fleming to help design Zimura's next trial—a screening trial with two arms to test different doses. The trial was set with a high hurdle, a confidence level of 95 percent, all the better to avoid an embarrassing Phase 3 like Fovista.

The Fovista disappointment changed David's perspective. He wanted to step back from day-to-day operations in what had become a very small company that was essentially in start-up mode again. Plus, he wanted to spend more time with his family and his two young sons. In the middle of the year, on July 1, David officially moved aside to let Glenn take over as CEO, in addition to being president. David maintained an eye on day-to-day operations, as his status on the company's board was elevated to executive chairman—typically a more hands-on role than chairman—while Glenn was also given a seat at the boardroom table. The increase in Glenn's responsibilities led David Carroll to step up from SVP of finance to assume Glenn's CFO position.

Gene therapy was the means to secure a broad array of assets, and as Ophthotech didn't build drugs from the ground up in labs, this meant scouring the planet for opportunities. It was the same approach Glenn used at the Medicines Company. "We created this global road map of the world of every available gene therapy product," Glenn explains. "We looked at universities, academics; we looked at early-stage companies."

"I literally traveled the world," Glenn reflects about building the gene therapy portfolio. "I spent eight days in China going to all these companies and institutions; went to Europe, to Germany, specifically Tübingen because there was a big eye center there; spent a lot of time in Belgium and London." Naturally, he canvassed the US, too. His business development team visited educational institutions on both coasts and pretty much anywhere in between where gene therapy was undergoing serious investigation. "We did a deal with the University of Massachusetts, with Dr. Gao, who's a leader in gene therapy and ophthalmology." Glenn also entered into agreements with the University of Pennsylvania and the University of Florida. "U Penn and U Florida," notes Glenn, "are really the innovators of gene therapy in ophthalmology with the design of capsids (protein shells that deliver genetic material)." He also considered looking for gene therapies to treat glaucoma but decided to stick to Ophthotech's original gambit at the back of the eye. All in all, Glenn and his team uncovered about eighty potential targets.

WHAT'S IN A NAME?

At the start of 2018, Kourous Rezaei, a highly respected retinal specialist, was promoted from SVP to become Ophthotech's chief medical officer. Throughout the year, Kourous helped Ophthotech continue its rapid tilt toward gene therapy while in the background, recruiting patients in the Zimura trials. These trials had an uncontrolled Phase 2a with 64 patients in combination with Lucentis and a double-masked controlled 2b trial with 286 patients of Zimura on its own to treat geographic atrophy (GA), an advanced stage of dry AMD that leads to further irreversible loss of vision. GA gets its odd name from the distinct patches of damaged or dead retinal tissue which resemble geographic maps in imagery scans. But there was another name that was bothering Glenn.

As the year passed, recruiting in trials picked up some speed, and there were more deals for gene therapy assets, but Glenn felt that although progress was being made on all fronts, something was holding the company back. Ophthotech, he believed, came with unnecessary baggage. The Fovista failure had stuck to it like gum on the sole of your shoe—or bird poop on your windshield—impeding efforts to move forward. "Everybody believed that anything from Ophthotech was bad," reflects Glenn. "We had no credibility." Changing direction to focus on gene therapy required not only acquiring new assets but also building a whole new brand. If Hollywood stars from Cary

Grant and Charlie Sheen to Whoopi Goldberg and Natalie Portman could find fame and fortune after changing their names, why not Ophthotech?

A habit at the Medicines Company was to emphasize precision and purpose in its branding by using names for drugs that had associations with Latin terminology, a practice rooted in scientific tradition. Glenn thought this approach would work for rebranding Ophthotech. To counter the credibility issue, his team settled on deriving a name from the Latin word for truth—*veritas*. With a little creativity and bringing ophthalmology into the picture—or at least the sound of *eye*—they came up with Iveric. The kicker was getting the NASDAQ to change the company's stock symbol to ISEE. Name it and claim it, as they say. Iveric Bio officially came into being on Wednesday, April 17, 2019, at the start of trading.

ANOTHER HORSE RACE

Although Glenn's team successfully narrowed down the target list of gene therapy products, they were encountering unexpected challenges. They were not seeing the responses in the preclinical studies that they'd hoped for. Something wasn't working in the drug delivery. A key mechanism for delivering the desired genetic material to a target cell is using a viral vector. After inserting a therapeutic gene into a virus, the virus surrounds the gene "like two firecrackers at the ends," as Glenn describes the setup. "When you inject it, the firecrackers go off; they release the gene." However, the process of manufacturing gene therapies was fraught with difficulties. It wasn't working as it should. Sparks weren't flying. And the end effect was like introducing an empty virus.

That wasn't the only worry of Glenn's. Despite the rebrand, Iveric's stock had yet to rebound. And Zimura had competition. A small company called Apellis, focused on developing drugs for autoimmune diseases, was also working on a complement inhibitor for GA. In August 2017, Apellis released results from its Phase 2 clinical trial with 246 patients, which showed that monthly intravitreal injections of its drug, APL-2, in six treatments, caused the rate of GA lesion growth to slow by 20 percent. After a year of monthly treatments, it was down by 47 percent. And even giving APL-2 once every two months brought a 33 percent decrease. Pretty impressive stuff for an untreatable disease. Enough for Kourous to take a deep look. Maybe complement inhibition really could work? Perhaps Iveric should shift its stance, as David constantly argued, and step up its game plan for Zimura.

Founded in Louisville, Kentucky, Apellis had a penchant for equine-themed nomenclature; its Phase 2 trial was called FILLY. With such positive results, the company galloped toward its two Phase 3 trials, named DERBY and OAKS, which received fast-track status from the FDA in mid-2018. For the folks at Iveric, this was a wake-up call. After being the first to perform an intravitreal injection with a complement inhibitor for dry AMD, they had lost time with Fovista, and since its failure, were primarily occupied with building their gene therapy portfolio. In a complete reversal of fortune compared to Eyetech's race with Genentech against Lucentis, Iveric found themselves now trailing behind Apellis.

Apellis's approach to GA was slightly different from Zimura: Its drug APL-2, which later became Syfovre, targets the C3 protein in the complement cascade, whereas Zimura is aimed at the C5 protein. In brief, C3 is like a central hub in the complement system where its three pathways converge. C5 is downstream from C3 and is part of the terminal pathway, which acts as a sort of executioner, disintegrating cells by rupturing their membranes. In essence, Syfovre provides a broader suppression of the complement system, and Zimura's mechanism is more focused.

In addition to the speed of Apellis's drug development, the company's attention to autoimmune disease and its successful trials were matched by its admirable fundraising. Its IPO in March 2019 garnered $113 million. Meanwhile, Iveric's stock dipped to just ninety-one cents in the middle of the year, bringing its market capitalization to just $44 million. A moment of reckoning was coming.

On October 28, 2019, Iveric released the results of Zimura's randomized and controlled Phase 2b trials. For drug doses of 2 mg and 4 mg, they were impressive: Over twelve months, both slowed the rate of GA growth by over 27 percent.

"Stop the presses!" Evelyn remembers the call she received from her chief medical officer, Kourous: "We're pivoting from gene therapy, and we got to set up a Phase 3 trial ASAP for the complement because it looks like this drug works." The younger child was the winner after all!

David felt vindicated. The clear lesson was that you should never favor a child. Treat them equally. He'd long suspected complement over activity could be a cause of dry AMD, and GA in particular. Back when he and Samir were originally looking at assets, the acquisition of the complement inhibitor brought to mind an unusual experience from his clinical practice days: "When I was in my thirties, I remember seeing a twenty-five-year-old female patient who had drusen." He explains the condition as "white and yellow spots at the back of the eye. It's really an early form of dry macular degeneration." He continues, "But it was shocking because a twenty-five-year-old should not have any signs of age-related disease." He wondered, "How could this possibly be?" Going through her medical records revealed that she had an autoimmune kidney disease. "It was called complement-mediated glomerulonephritis, a well-known condition. Basically, a stimulation of the complement portion of the immune system to cause kidney damage." Although David was unclear about all the processes involved, he saw a connection: "At least to me, this was the first evidence that the complement system could be involved in macular degeneration." Since that time, there had been a wealth of epidemiology and genetics linking the complement system to AMD.

David and Kourous took the data to Wiley Chambers at the FDA. With his input, they came up with a design for a Phase 3 trial. "We were off to the races," says Glenn. "The stock responded well; it went up from a buck to four dollars. We started to raise money. We did a private placement. The momentum picked up. There was interest from Wall Street."

"The plan was to get things up and running in January," according to Evelyn, who knew they needed to make up for lost time. "The protocols were written over the Christmas holidays." By the end of February 2020, they were already shipping the drug out to multiple sites. "Everything was set up," says Glenn proudly. "We were going to start the trial in early March."

COVID STRIKES—AND SAVES THE DAY

"This is going to sound crazy," warns Glenn, "but COVID saved the company."

Glenn sent a team consisting of Iveric's chief medical officer, Kourous Rezaei, vice president of investor relations, Kathy Galante, chief financial officer, Dave Carroll, and chief operating officer, Keith Westby, to the Cowen and Company's Fortieth Annual Health Care Conference at the Boston Marriott. It was an investor gathering, and on March 4, Iveric did a presentation. "We get a note at the end of the week," recalls Glenn, "that a number of people had got sick. We know this virus thing was going around."

Indeed, just a few days earlier, a similar conference in Boston became a super-spreader event. It took a while for health researchers to determine this, but Channel 7 in Boston reported months later, "Boston Biotech conference led to 333,000 COVID-19 cases across US, genetic fingerprinting shows." *The New York Times*, covering the incident, said, "The virus strains spread to at least 29 states. They were found in Australia, Sweden, and Slovakia." The publication claimed that at the time of the event, only thirty coronavirus infections had been confirmed in the United States.

"You know what? Don't come into the office. Take the week off; work from home," Glenn told Dave, Kathy, Keith, and Kourous upon their return. "They got pissed at me. They said, 'I've got a lot to do.'" But they followed orders, and fortunately, none of them became ill. It was increasingly apparent that COVID-19 infections in the US were following the patterns established elsewhere in the world and that the whole situation was rapidly deteriorating.

Even before the federal government declared an emergency and started issuing travel bans, Glenn took action. By the end of the first week in March, Glenn told his team, "Don't start the trial now. Let's pause it." To ensure there were no inappropriate injections, Glenn had Keith arrange for all the doses to be returned from the test sites where the drug had been distributed. The company issued an SEC 8-K notification, warning shareholders that a "material event" was taking place: "We sent out a press release. Whatever the stock was trading at, we got killed."

After conferring with some other CEOs, Glenn decided by the second week of March to send out a note to the company saying, "Due to the uncertainty and with an abundance of caution, why don't we all work from home for the next two weeks. At the end of March, we'll get some clarity on this." He was ahead of New York Governor Mario Cuomo by several days, as New York State mandated working from home for nonessential jobs starting on March 20. Of course, the end of the month came and went without anyone returning to the office.

Glenn considered the new remote working model a challenge to be solved: "I thought long and hard about how to do this." He realized the main problem to overcome was isolation, ensuring people kept in touch. "We put in communication plans. We put in a buddy system. I had weekly town halls," says Glenn of the efforts. "We made sure that I had implemented a Monday morning and Friday morning touch-base with the leadership team." The communication went beyond business concerns: "We started talking about families and how they're dealing with everything." Glenn declared, "When I say it saved us, it bonded the company in a way that was so unique."

David was also active. He gave the company Zoom presentations on the latest COVID-19 developments. Summarizing the most up-to-date medical information on the virus, what people should be thinking about, and how best to protect themselves. As vaccines came on the scene, he kept everyone posted on their development. "He gave the most amazing presentations at the height of the pandemic," recalls Evelyn. "People could level-set, feel at ease; it calmed them."

Meanwhile, Glenn also pondered how to keep the business running. He asked Keith and Evelyn to consult with their teams and find out:

"How do we restart this trial in this period when people are dying and our patients are old and have comorbidities?" Evelyn was able to put the information garnered from David's lectures to use. With Evelyn's guidance, the company went on a personal protective equipment, or PPE, spending spree. "We bought thousands and thousands of masks. We bought gloves, bought face shields. Twenty-four cases of Clorox wipes," Glenn recollects. With no one at the office, Glenn had everything shipped to his house. It wound up on his porch waiting to get wiped down. His daughter was alarmed. "Dad, you've got to take that in!" she exclaimed. "That's like gold sitting on the front porch!"

Glenn's five thousand N95 masks formed the foundation of a plan. Beyond the PPE, his team conjured up a protocol for getting patients to doctors' clinics to receive their shots. "We hired limo services—with single, high-quality drivers. We sent them our masks and Clorox wipes," he explains. "Their job was to pick the person up with gloves, with masks, with face shields, and make sure the car is wiped down." Evelyn also put in place an intricate program to keep patients happy while en route: She procured cutting boards and put them, plus sandwich ingredients, in Iveric-branded lunch bags. Patients could make their own lunch, free from contact with anyone else. These kits came along with blankets for warmth and security. "So as the patient was in the car, they had their own lunch; they had their blanket; they had their personal protection," says Glenn proudly. When they got to the doctor's office or clinic, they would find all the furniture arranged in a way that minimized contact and provided the most safety during the procedure, something that the Iveric team had instructed the medical personnel how best to do. Everything was up and running by August. "Our patient retention rate was 95 percent," recounts Glenn. An impressive figure even when there isn't a pandemic.

"To Evelyn's credit, and the team's credit, and the docs' credit," Glenn acknowledges, "we were able to close the gap on Apellis." As Glenn sees it, Apellis perhaps wasn't so fortunate, apparently having problems losing patients during COVID as well as possibly experiencing manufacturing difficulties. "We started three years behind. In the end, when we got to NDA and approval, we closed the gap to six months." Along the way, Iveric picked up some time with the first trial, and doing Phase 3 during the height of COVID gained them more than a year. A minor hiccup occurred filing for a special protocol assessment (SPA), but once that was smoothed out, they were back on track, in the fast lane. Wall Street duly noted the astonishing progress, and through a heavily oversubscribed secondary offering, Glenn was able to raise money for commercialization. Finally, after getting the data in 2022, they were able to file the NDA in a record three months. Looking back at this impressive teamwork, Glenn says simply, "It was brilliant."

ENDPOINT MET

"Iveric Bio's strong management team has evolved to the point where there is no longer a need for an executive chair," stated Dr. David Guyer. "After fifteen years on the board, I feel that this is a good departure point such that I can return to my passion as a venture capitalist." Thus read the company's press release issued on April 5, 2021. David would end his tenure at the conclusion of the annual stockholders' meeting on May 21. After that, he was back at SV Health Investors while still serving as a senior advisor to Iveric.

At this time, Pravin Dugel who joined Iveric as EVP in April 2020, became president. Pravin's deep experience as a leading investigator in over one hundred clinical trials would help ensure clinical progress.

Even though Glenn was able to raise funds to commercialize Zimura, around the middle of 2022, the scale of this project started to dawn on him: "If this thing gets approved, it's bigger than us, and there's no way that we can do it on our own." His idea was to sell the company, and after some discussion, the board was, it seemed, behind it.

The first part of the NDA was submitted to the FDA in November. Just two weeks later the FDA awarded Zimura a "breakthrough therapy" designation, meaning it was intended to treat a serious unmet medical need, and its regulatory review could be accelerated. Another round of fundraising ensued, and 13.35 million shares of common stock were offered. With all the positive news of the last few years, the share price was a healthy $22.50, which comes to a total of a cool $300 million. Despite the momentum, Glenn was convinced success required more than money; it needed a partner with worldwide reach. Before the year was done, Glenn quietly approached the global investment and advisory firm Centerview, who were very attuned to the ambient buzz of the biotech market.

By the first quarter of 2023, it appeared that Iveric was on the radar of a significant number of potential strategic partners. Numerous meetings ensued. The Japanese giant Astellas was very interested. By the end of April, a deal was negotiated. For a company that not too long ago was trading at less than a dollar, the offer of forty dollars per share in cash—$5.9 billion in all (a 64 percent premium on its current share price)—was an offer that no one in their right mind would refuse.

For Astellas, it was a chance to build its portfolio in one of its five key areas of focus: blindness and regeneration. Although Astellas took some of Iveric's gene therapy programs, and the University of Pennsylvania initiative went to a company formed by the Foundation Fighting Blindness, there's no doubt that the C5 complement inhibitor, Zimura, was the reason for Iveric's huge sale.

IN HINDSIGHT

Samir and David's initial business plan of bringing in two assets in 2007 was successful. It just took a little longer, involved only the second asset and a big downturn on the way. But they got there and won big in the end.

Don't look for Zimura if you or a loved one need treatment for dry AMD. After approval by the FDA in August 2023, the drug's name was changed from Zimura to Izervay.

Changing a name, whether from Zimura to Izervay or Ophthotech to Iveric, may increase the appeal of a drug or a company, but it's what lies beneath that's truly significant. For Glenn, that comes down to the people whom he believed in and who believed in the company. "Iveric, for me, was one of the hardest things I've done. We were down and out, with a $39 million market capitalization, a failed company in September 2019. And we sold it for $6 billion." Reflecting on this, he says, "It took that whole team, together. Nobody left. I mean, I lost two people out of the original twenty-eight; they stayed through COVID to help."

"The finish line for me," Evelyn says, "is that the drug worked in getting FDA approval. That for me was huge because I'm an optimist. I could have left. I wanted to finish on top. I did not want to leave after ten years with a massively failed drug." Although some friends had implored her to go, asking her, "Why are you staying there? The company's a dog." She is grateful for seeing it through. "For me, getting the drug on the market to treat dry AMD—that meant the world to me. After sixteen years—sixteen long, arduous, roller-coaster years—but at the end, there's a drug out there for patients, to help improve patients' lives." For the second time, a drug for a previously untreatable disease! And the sale? "Just a bonus," Evelyn adds. "Icing. A cherry on the top. Like, oh my God, this is even better!"

For David and Samir, the approval of Zimura/Izervay and the sale of the company was validation. At the very beginning, they picked an incredibly valuable asset, one that could provide relief to the 200 million people around the world suffering from dry AMD.

"We had people in business development that were scouring the globe to see what else was out there," Evelyn says of the final irony of Iveric's sale. "And meanwhile, we had the winner all along—sitting over a decade in our possession."

In the end, David and Samir had been right the whole time. The market's reaction to Fovista's failure was blind to the reality that all of Ophthotech's eggs weren't in one basket. Was it reasonable to expect the company would be right 100 percent of the time? Who in biotech can claim that?

David and Samir's second coin toss came up heads. Big time—to the tune of $6 billion.

Chapter 11

THIRD TIME'S A CHARM

"The grass is always greener in venture capital. There's always something exciting happening," remarks David about his return to SV Health Investors in 2021. But rather than surfing from board to board across multiple companies, David remained single-minded: "I really like smaller companies, building them. EyeBio was started immediately—almost the same day I left Iveric. It just wasn't official until the money was in."

"David called us and said he'd like to do it again," recalls Dame Kate Bingham, SV's London-based managing partner who co-leads the firm's biotech franchise. Kate had just earned her royally bestowed honorific as chair of the UK vaccine task force, reporting directly to Prime Minister Boris Johnson, while heading a team of world-class experts to source and produce COVID-19 vaccines and help their country be the first Western country to vaccinate its population. "And I was trying to extricate myself from government at that point," she remembers. "I put David onto my partner and said, 'You better talk about the science to him.'"

Everyone at SV quickly understood that David wanted to follow a similar model to Ophthotech and Eyetech—one that focused on search and development, rather than creating a company with in-house labs to perform underlying research and discovery work. He would figure out the areas of biology that are the most useful and interesting, then look for candidate molecules to in-license, which would be optimized and taken into clinical trials. "So, the first step was to find the assets," stated David. "The assets available drive the process."

Lucentis and other anti-VEGF therapies have had a profound impact on patient health, but their effect isn't total. They prevent many people from going blind, but they aren't cures for age-related macular degeneration and diabetic macular edema. The disease doesn't disappear. Over time, the benefit of the drugs diminishes. After five years, 50 percent of patients go back to baseline. Not only that, around 60 percent of patients treated with current therapies have suboptimal outcomes, and 30 percent still have active disease. Anti-VEGF treatments have essentially hit an efficacy ceiling. The need to do better is still urgent.

Several retinal conditions are characterized by both inflammation and breakdown of the blood-retinal barrier (BRB), a dynamic barrier that controls the passage of ions, molecules, and fluids from the bloodstream into the inner retina. Breakdowns result in vascular permeability and leakage into the neighboring retinal tissue. This seepage is a known risk factor for retinal diseases including DME and neovascular age-related macular degeneration (better known as "wet AMD"). With this in mind, David set about looking for a mechanism of action that might help those 60 percent of patients who aren't benefitting fully from anti-VEGF drugs and the 30 percent who, in reality, aren't experiencing any response at all.

"Show me every business plan you rejected over the last year and a half in ophthalmology," was David's call to action back on board at SV. He was looking for the molecule at the center of a business proposal that showed promise but may have been passed over for ancillary reasons. (Perhaps the market potential was unclear, the science was not well understood, the management team was not complete, or the capital requirements were deemed excessive.) His focus was on what the asset does. There were many questions at the front of his mind: Is that something we could work with? Could it be a great drug? Is the affinity high? Does it work? What's the likelihood it'll work in this disease? Is it easy to manufacture? David summarizes, "It's a very high hurdle to get a molecule like that. We looked at hundreds of assets. At the end of the day, we're going to bring in two or three assets to the company."

One that caught David's attention was a molecule, soon to be assigned the moniker Restoret (EYE103) by David's team, from a private company called AntlerA. After David unearthed it in a pile of discarded business plans, it was brought to his consideration by Alex Badamchi-Zadeh, a key member of SV's investment team.

The Bay Area–based AntlerA had been on the radar of several VC firms, but despite having a great team of scientists producing stellar work under the leadership of Somasekar (Sekar) Seshagiri—a veteran genomics expert who spent over two decades at Genentech—the investment consensus was the company didn't possess clinical development expertise.

Nevertheless, Restoret (EYE103), in David's view, was an exciting molecule. It was a Wnt agonist. Jointly discovered in the early 1980s by Roel Nusse, who received the Breakthrough Prize in Life Sciences for his work, and the Nobel laureates J. Michael Bishop and Harold Varmus, the latter of which became the director of the National Institutes of Health and the National Cancer Institute, the Wnt signaling pathways are involved in a wide range of biological phenomena. What intrigued David was the possibility of using Restoret (EYE103) as an anti-permeability agent; it had the potential to stop blood vessels from leaking. Here was a molecule that could possibly make excess fluid go away and restore the retinal barrier, whose breakdown is a fundamental part of the disease. Together these approaches could be a one-two punch for retinal diseases. He realized it was time to talk to his old friend Tony Adamis.

"David and I had always stayed in touch," recounts Tony. "He had asked me to join the board of Iveric, but I was prohibited when I was at Genentech.

The pair had last worked together at Eyetech. Following the transition that occurred after the sale to OSI, they parted ways. Tony took a few members of the Eyetech team, including Dave Shima, and cofounded Jerini Ophthalmic, a wholly-owned, independent US subsidiary of the

German company, Jerini, AG. Not long after, Jerini was sold to Shire, a UK firm that hopped the pond and set up headquarters in Massachusetts before being gobbled up by the Japanese conglomerate Takeda in 2019. Genentech made overtures to Tony while he was at Jerini, but he was reluctant to work for such a giant company. But once Jerini became part of a much larger organization, Tony accepted an invitation to Genentech's West Coast campus. If nothing else, it would be an opportunity to say hi to Napoleone Ferrara. "I went out there and they wowed me," Tony reflects. "On the flight back, I was thinking, 'How am I going to convince my wife to move to California?'" But after years in Boston and New York, she was readily seduced by the charms of the Bay Area. "It wasn't a hard sell."

In 2009, Tony became Genentech's global head of Ophthalmology. "It was a great job," says Tony. "Genentech had just been acquired by Roche, and they really wanted to invest in ophthalmology. I loved it." Tony quickly found he had an appetite for more, and he took on all the additional responsibilities offered to him by his boss: "Basically, I ran everything but oncology. I had immunology, infectious disease, neurology, everything." This meant running all the clinical trials for those indications. "I had a huge portfolio of drugs, a global team. I had a wonderful team of people around the world. There were people in China, in London, and in Basel, Switzerland. I would fly around the world and meet with those teams and help lead the development of all the drugs." If that wasn't enough, his duties also included working with the early discovery teams to come up with new drugs. "One of them was Vabysmo. Now it's a very important drug in ophthalmology." The medication's mechanism may allow some retinal disease patients to receive less frequent anti-VEGF injections. Since the development of Macugen and Lucentis, it's clear people would rather get a needle in the eye than go blind. Still, getting a shot in the eye is far from pleasant. Who doesn't want to reduce the number of injections they need to receive? The popularity of Vabysmo has led to sales of over $4 billion annually. But by 2021, Tony had reached a natural separation point. "I learned an awful lot about other disease areas besides ophthalmology and also got to grow ophthalmology and was able to introduce new therapies." After having brought fourteen drugs to approval across thirty-two diseases over the course of his career, he stepped away from Genentech and moved to Florida. Just in time to assist David.

"As soon as I finished in the summer of 2021, literally, the first call I got was David." The two friends discussed the interesting AntlerA molecule. The idea of a Wnt agonist for ophthalmology was intriguing. "What do you think?" David asked Tony. "Do you want to be involved?"

Tony shared his friend's enthusiasm. "I looked into it, and it was a really exciting molecule, a new pathway. Potentially it could be an important drug."

Together the duo, David as CEO and Tony as CSO, answered Kate's most important question: "Is there a company to build here?"

Summing up their analysis, Tony says, "It was the bringing in of Restoret (EYE103) that was the catalyst for starting and funding EyeBio."

WNT—THE AGONIST AND THE ECSTASY

You are built of water. It's in your blood. Depending on your level of hydration, the ubiquitous liquid comprises 80 to 85 percent of the blood circulating through your body. But it's water that kills you eventually. As you advance in years, just like an old building, your body's internal plumbing starts to leak. Aging brings on a failure of the vascular system. Edema is the medical term for the accumulation of excess fluid. When it happens in your heart, kidney, or liver, that's the end of you. In the back of the eye, you go blind. But if you could drive your embryonic systems—the parts of you constructed when you were still a fetus—to restore tissue, maybe you can reverse the effects of aging.

The Wnt/β-catenin signaling pathway plays a role in fetal vascular development, as well as adult stem cell maintenance, so much of the early investigation into the Wnt pathway focused on developing antiaging remedies. Activation of Wnt signaling promotes tissue repair and regeneration which declines with age.

The Wnt pathway is a very complex system of cascading events. At the heart of this process, a family of proteins is brought together on the surface of a cell. This gathering is orchestrated by a Norrin, a small protein with a special structure that allows it to bind specifically to certain receptors, making it a highly effective signaling molecule. When the Norrin successfully draws these proteins together, it causes an activation, sending a signal downstream. In essence, something on the outside of a cell triggers the release of an internal compound, β-catenin, which regulates the formation and stabilization of blood vessels. Included in this process is the transcription of the genes responsible for the development and maintenance of the blood-retina barrier.

The challenge for biotech was to recreate the Norrin synthetically, fabricating a molecule known as a Norrin-mimetic. It had been attempted numerous times without success. A convoluted procedure, achieving it required a leap forward in molecular engineering and manufacturing. "There are many Wnts," explains Tony. "The specific Wnt we are addressing with Restoret (EYE103) is FZD4/LRP5, which is expressed only on the blood vessels feeding the retina. This is the same Wnt addressed by Norrin."

Luckily, Kate shared David and Tony's enthusiasm. Working with an agonist instead of a molecule that blocked activity, had some advantages. "It's enhancing a signal that's already there," she notes, "and that means you can put in a much smaller amount." Although she was referring to the dosage of the potential drug, her remark also applied to the size of the investment required at this early stage. When SV contacted AntlerA, they were ready to have an entirely different conversation from their previous ones a year earlier.

Speaking with Sekar Seshagiri, David felt an instant rapport with the AntlerA CEO, and the feelings were mutual: "He knew some of the stuff Tony and I had done before." David also felt sympathy for his situation. "His team was continuing to struggle to raise money in a very tough market," David remembers. What David proposed was an entirely different approach. Instead of trying to find investors to support all of AntlerA's platform, why not license Restoret (EYE103) to EyeBio? Not only would this ease some of AntlerA's financial headaches but also enable David and Tony to pursue a much bigger prize. Whereas AntlerA initially focused on using Restoret (EYE103) to treat a hereditary eye condition called FEVR (familial exudative vitreoretinopathy), a rare disease with fewer than two hundred thousand patients in the US, EyeBio would expand the focus to include DME and wet AMD, conditions that are many orders of magnitude bigger. For David and Tony, this was extremely familiar territory; for AntlerA tackling this would be more difficult. Sekar immediately understood the appeal.

By June 2021, it all was coming together. SV provided an initial $4 million of seed money, enough to in-license EyeBio's first asset and run a series of toxicity tests, which went smoothly. The next step was to test the molecule in humans. And put some humans in an office, even if it was a virtual one.

LONDON CALLING

As SV was a limited partnership based in the UK, to simplify funding requirements, it made the most sense for EyeBio to be a UK company. "I needed a UK general manager," muses David about staffing the EyeBio headquarters on the other side of the pond where Kate was installed as chairman of its board. "But I hadn't worked with anybody in the UK."

Luckily, a fortuitous cascade of voice signaling followed Kate's departure from the UK vaccine task force. Her place at its head was filled by Dr. Clive Dix, an old friend of Kate's who was also chairman of Touchlight, a British biotech firm focused on developing DNA-based genetic medicines. Touchlight had just undergone a transformation following an extensive round of fundraising. The small company shifted direction, deciding to concentrate on manufacturing rather than development.

The change left Sarah Milsom, the firm's vice president of translation, feeling unsettled. She'd told Dix, and he asked her to call him when she was ready for something new.

"I did," says Sarah, looking back on her move. "And he said, 'Look, I'm flat out with the vaccine task force, but Kate Bingham knows everybody and everything. I'll introduce you and go speak to her." When Sarah called Kate, she didn't have anything on hand but assured Sarah she'd come back to her when something popped up.

True to her word, about two weeks later, Sarah's phone rang. A couple of possibilities had appeared, including this new SV start-up, EyeBio. "And kindly, she and one other person from SV interviewed me," recalls Sarah. But despite the warm feelings, they left her with the impression that meeting David was unlikely to lead to anything further, saying, "By the way, David doesn't hire anybody he hasn't worked with before. It's just sort of his nature and paranoia about working with strangers." Still, Sarah thought she had nothing to lose. She had read about David and was keen to speak to someone with his track record. At the very least, it would be practice for future interviews.

To Sarah's surprise, when they met, she and David got along extremely well. Not only was she comfortable informing him about her experience with preclinical work, in- and out-licensing, and fundraising, but she was also upfront about her lack of experience with clinical trials, which clearly would be the immediate focus of EyeBio. The pair formed a bond over their mutual sense of paranoia and obsessive-compulsive behaviors. "I told him that I used to play a game in the car as a child where I would imagine all possible scenarios for an accident and how I would get out of them alive," says Sarah, replaying their conversation. "I think he liked that..." The result: He hired her.

Echoing David's overture to Evelyn at the dawn of Ophthotech, he told Sarah that anything she didn't already know, he would teach her or find someone who could. The short time it took for David to explain that was for Sarah the single most important developmental talk in her career. It made her realize she didn't need to know everything. What was important was knowing when to ask for help and then getting the best advice. It's a dictum she's followed ever since. In October 2021, she officially became employee number two. And besides that, in the future, every other employee except the yet-to-be-hired chief medical officer would report to her. Sarah would be David's sole report on the business side. The operational build of the company, the preclinical development, manufacturing, finance, legal, and HR were all hers.

Looking back, Sarah feels she couldn't have picked a better learning experience. "David's an incredible teacher and is entirely convinced of the view that if someone has sufficient intelligence, it doesn't matter what they know or don't know; nothing's really that hard. 'Just go and talk to people, build a plan, and come back and talk to me about it or talk to me before you do it.' With this simple instruction, he empowered me to be the executive he wanted. This instruction enabled me to tackle this terrifying role, one decision at a time." And David felt Sarah was a quick learner, a little obsessive, and a touch paranoid—plus a very hard worker—just like him. They clicked.

A BETTER MOUSETRAP

The business side of EyeBio effectively delegated, David turned his attention to the science; he needed a chief medical officer—and fast. Unlike taking a chance on someone unknown, as he did with Sarah, David already knew the right guy for the job: the chairman of the Department of Ophthalmology at Rutgers Robert Wood Johnson Medical School, Jonathan Prenner. In fact, not only had he known the Princeton, New Jersey–based doctor for almost two decades, he'd already offered him a job before. Jon had turned down David's previous proposition to be CMO at Iveric, but in hindsight, after the company's $6 billion sale to Astellas, David thought Jon may be ready now. It was certainly worth trying to woo him one more time.

The relationship between the two eye doctors went all the way back to when Jon was a retinal fellow participating in the Macugen trials in the early 2000s. Jon remembers those pioneering days of intravitreal injections, before a simple, straightforward method became routine: "I had a *Wall Street Journal* reporter come and watch me give one of my first injections. It was so novel." Jon's lucky patient was a former scientist at Los Alamos, who didn't mind being treated in front of a member of the press. "It was incredible." In addition to embracing the therapeutic future of retinal treatment, Jon witnessed the passing of the old ways. "I actually performed thermal laser of the macula," he jokes. "I'm probably the last person who was trained to do that procedure."

As well as his wealth of experience, Jon also brought the perspective of a practicing retinal specialist to the role of CMO. "I have a clinical practice," explains Jon. "I'm in the office seeing patients. I get to give that kind of perspective. And David and Tony recognized that." Jon experienced an additional benefit to the company being centered in London. Surprisingly the transatlantic time difference was in Jon's favor: "It worked out well because of surgeon's hours. I'm up early and can talk to the team at five o'clock in the morning my time. No problem."

Jon had all the attributes David liked: world-class expertise (as one of the top retinal surgeons in the world), low ego, and total transparency. Jon came on board right after Sarah. In the meantime, Jon had reached out to Matt Feinsod, Eyetech's SVP of strategy and product development to get up to speed and was told by Matt, "Jobs 1-10 on your to-do list are patient safety." Although as a contractor, Jon technically wasn't employee number three, this didn't diminish his commitment. "As CMO, my primary responsibility—and I take this extremely seriously—is 'protect the patients.' Everyone else has other responsibilities. I'm the only one who has that charge."

With safety in mind, Jon recognized being at a small biotech start-up probably gave him more latitude in designing clinical trials than at a large pharmaceutical company. Also, he enjoyed Tony and David's hands-off management style, which consisted of working with people they trust and giving them white space. "And not have eleven meetings a day and pick apart every word," Jon adds, noting the environment was "very progressive." But the extra freedom comes with great responsibility. "The worst thing that can happen when you're an early-phase company is to get a false negative," he explains. "You have a real drug candidate that could help people, and you test it in a way that winds up giving you a falsely negative result." An event that has sunk many biotech start-ups. Jon continues, "You have to give yourself the opportunity to demonstrate a true positive response [seeing an effect in patients that could only be explained by the candidate working] because if you want to accelerate the program and secure funding, then you really need to have data that people can say, 'Ah, this does work.' And creating a design that allows you to navigate the tension between seeing a true positive and avoiding a false negative takes a lot of creativity."

Jon envisioned a unique setup, a two-part Phase 1b/2a trial. The first part was an open-label multiple ascending dose (MAD) component, meaning four cohorts of patients, staggered at weekly intervals, would each receive increasingly larger doses of Restoret (EYE103). The second phase was a dose-finding trial. The primary goal here was to test the efficacy of the molecule. Eventually, like all drug candidates, Restoret (EYE103) would need to go through a rigorous process of two controlled, randomized Phase 3 trials to achieve FDA approval.

The full name of the trial was to be "Anti-Permeability Mechanism and Age-Related Ocular Neovascularization Evaluation," more smoothly referred to by its acronym AMARONE. No doubt the reference to the classic Italian wine from the Valpolicella region made with slightly dried grapes, possessing an intense red color, and a full, velvety, although slightly bitter, flavor was designed to reflect David's epicurean enthusiasm. "If you're in the test kitchen with someone like me," reflects Jon of his trial design "who comes up with something totally different, and then to have David say, 'Yeah that makes sense. Let's do that.' It shows he's iconoclastic." According to Jon, David doesn't adhere to the way things have been done in the past: "If you have a better mousetrap, David wants to do that instead. As long as it doesn't put patients at risk and it's okay with regulatory authorities, he's on board with trying something new. And that's what has made EyeBio so successful and so fun." Ultimately, when the AMARONE data was publicly presented just over two years later, at the Macular Society Meeting on February 8, 2024, Jon's tinkering proved to be a recipe for apparent success.

IMPATIENCE IS A VIRTUE, TOO

SV's $4 million in seed financing was sufficient to set up the trial. Now, serious money to run a substantially sized trial needed to be raised. SV had already put feelers out in the venture world to gather support for a Series A investment round. But once again, the general financial picture for the biotech world was grim. "We started up EyeBio in just about the worst period of biotech funding there has ever been," Jon reflects.

It was a verdict that Srini Akkaraju concurred with. In Srini's view, following the pandemic, there was an investment wave in biotech powered by, as he put it, "the hype and hysteria of Moderna." But after cresting in early 2021, "it went down and continued to go down relentlessly for several years." Since his encounter with Eyetech, on his first day at JP Morgan in 2001, Srini has witnessed plenty of ups and downs. Still, he characterized the environment commencing just before EyeBio's Series A round as dire: "[It was] the longest and deepest down cycle that I've personally experienced as a biotech investor for over twenty-four years."

For the past eight of those years, Srini has helmed Samsara BioCapital, headquartered in Silicon Valley. As a fledgling firm in 2017, it invested heavily in Ophthotech during its IPO and then in Iveric, when the first positive data on the complement inhibitor came out. Srini started his company, Samsara, after stints at New Leaf Venture Partners and Sofinnova Venture, which followed his time at Panorama Capital, spun off from JP Morgan in 2006. Over the years, he's invested in a wide range of therapies for a broad spectrum of medical conditions, but eye disease has remained an area of interest.

Samsara had also been watching AntlerA and had discussions with Sekar Seshagiri but eventually reached the same conclusion as other venture firms. When SV approached Srini to join the Series A syndicate, he was already familiar with Restoret (EYE103), and knowing that it was going into the hands of David and Tony gave him the confidence that the asset's clinical development would be expertly managed. Samsara was in.

Finding other firms to join the syndicate wasn't quite so straightforward. Not only was the biotech environment dour, but interest in ophthalmology was particularly sour. A company called Kodiak Sciences, also focused on retinal disease, had left a bad taste in investors' mouths after an enthusiastically promoted IPO at the end of 2020 drove the company's stock price to a peak of $169.98 in January 2021, and following the announcement that its drug failed to match Eylea's efficacy in a Phase 2b/3 trial, its stock plummeted to $4.90 in May of the next year. Consequently, the general appetite for risk evaporated.

Sarah remembers the time as being particularly tricky for EyeBio: "This was not the time to be seeking venture investment in novel, preclinical assets. Everyone thought it was risky because the mechanism of action was not validated in clinical trials," says Sarah. "David is laser focused on acceleration. When you think about the Macugen story, a lot of the value in that business was their clear position as first to market. Even as better data started to emerge from the next generation anti-VEGF assets, the lead position was very important." Money often acts as an accelerant. But in tough markets, it's difficult to convince investors to step on the gas. Sarah was accutely aware of the dilemma. "Winning is about timing as much as it is about clinical data. A plan to win has to be as fast as possible."

Despite its supreme importance, the asset isn't the only thing investors consider. Jon sees the ordeal this way: "When you raise money, a lot of it's about what the asset is, what drug candidate do you have? There is asset risk: Is the thing going to work? There's market risk: is there enough of a need for it? And a lot of it's about the team. You can have a great asset—bad team—you're not getting anywhere close to the finish line. But we never had to worry about the team. It was not a normal start-up."

From Jon's perspective, the team more than compensated for any uncertainty around the asset. "EyeBio had David. And Tony Adamis, at his last job, he had many people reporting to him at Genentech! They're experienced; they've sold multiple companies. They're the founders of the space and created an approximately $22 billion annual market. It's very different when you have those kind of credentials behind you. That's a very atypical founder experience. Raising money is way better when you have those guys on the Zoom with you!"

By Thanksgiving 2021, a syndicate was on the verge of coming together. However, when it came to signing contracts, a Boston-based investment firm went silent. "We couldn't get hold of them," recalls Sarah. "Suddenly, we heard they were out. They cited a decision to invest only in clinical-stage assets due to the funding environment." This was particularly unnerving. "It was the most dreaded response we could have received," explains Sarah, "as it reinforced a barrier to investment that was not easy to move."

Undeterred, the small group pitched to around thirty-five different investors. The final contributions to the round came from Jeito Capital, an investment fund based in Paris and MRL Ventures Fund, the venture arm of Merck & Co., Inc. (Rahway, New Jersey, USA). By February 2022 SV, Samsara, Jeito, and MRL, were willing to commit $65 million. All that remained was to finalize the paperwork.

"When we got the syndicate together," explains Sarah, "David was like, 'Alright, we've got the first pass of the legal agreement. I don't want you to sleep until this is done.'" Sarah responded, "Why? It's fine. It's just going to take the time it takes." But, no, David was firm. He explained the current urgency was based on past experience; he'd been in Sarah's shoes before. "Marty Glick did this to me," he said, casting his mind back to the beginning of Eyetech. "When I started my first company, he pushed and pushed and pushed and pushed and pushed and said, 'You've got to close it. Now you've got it on the table. You close it; you close it!'" Just like Sarah, he was resistant at first, but he followed through. "We closed it. And the next day was 9/11. Had we not closed it, we would've never secured that financing. We wouldn't have got financing for another six to twelve months." Impressed but still nonplussed, Sarah said, "Okay, fine, you know about these things." A flurry of activity followed. "We went for it," she says. "We pushed everybody as hard as we could. We closed the financing. The next day Russia declared war on Ukraine. Which made the whole market even worse."

After she recovered from the frantic deal closure, Sarah woke up to a shocking reality. "It was utterly terrifying," she says, reliving the feeling. "Someone gave me a budget of spending millions a month!" She'd never dealt with this level of monetary responsibility, leaving her previous post just as the company had reached solid financial ground. Touchlight's early funding was modest, largely provided via the UK government's Enterprise Investment Scheme, which, as Sarah explains, "is sort of dribs and drabs from Formula One race drivers and soccer players seeking tax-efficient moon shots."

TRIALS AND CELEBRATIONS

With the money to go forward, the first hurdle to clear was ensuring the drug supply for the trials. EyeBio secured a couple of part-time advisors as team members (announced in a press release on March 6, 2023): Mike Davies, a CMC manufacturing expert who was VP of protein sciences at F-Star, worked for Lonza for sixteen years, and was familiar with developing complex molecules, and Paul Stephens, the former head of antibody biology at UCB and a biochemist with extensive experience in antibody development and discovery. Mike and Paul's experience helped the team avoid any problems and kept the momentum going. "Had it not been for these two," says Sarah, "we would not have had that kind of speed." EyeBio brought Paul on as SVP biology and Mike on board to serve as chief technical officer. Also mentioned in the press release, David brought members from his teams at Eyetech and Ophthotech, including Loni da Silva as chief regulatory officer and Eric Ng as SVP biology.

As the company grew, all the various pieces for the trial started falling into place, the March 6, press release duly noted the filing an Investigational New Drug (IND) application, which the FDA must approve before any human trials can commence, went smoothly, allowing Jon to reach out to his network of retinal specialists to start filling in the ranks of investigators.

While preparation for the Restoret (EYE103) trial remained in the foreground, in the background, the global search for the second asset continued. As Tony's team, which included Eric Ng as SVP Biology, uncovered something interesting, Jon, through his network, was also homing in on a potentially interesting molecule. Although coming from different directions, they both zeroed in on the same candidate. In October 2022, EyeBio acquired its second asset.

As 2022 rolled into 2023, with the investigators in place, recruitment commenced. On June 14, 2023, the first patient received an injection of Restoret (EYE103) (Announced in a press release on 6/14/2023). A week later, it was time to check if there were any immediate adverse effects. Jon received a text from a colleague, a world-renowned retina specialist: "Holy shit! This thing works!"

The doctor was astounded by the rapid improvement of the patient both in gaining vision and in imaging, something that almost never happens on its own. He sent pictures to Jon showing the change. Something was clearly happening in the back of the eye. And this doctor wasn't alone—Jon started to receive similarly enthusiastic text messages from other retinal specialists. They were witnessing significant fluid resolution in some patients, meaning the patient's eyes were no longer leaking. Of course, these are very early findings and only large-scale Phase 3 randomized, controlled clinical trials can accurately determine the potential efficacy and safety of a drug.

Unlike other organs in the body, doctors can see right into patients' eyes. Using optical coherence tomography (OTC), ophthalmologists beam light into the eye to take pictures that reveal cross-sections of the retina. The images produced readily measure and map the retina's thickness, or amount of swelling in the retina, so it's very easy to see changes—not something you can do when testing drugs in the pancreas, liver, or anywhere else. Jon explains, "In the eye, you can look into the tissue architecture directly and observe the very tissue that you are trying to treat. I could see exactly what's happening." Even though the study was small, approximately 30 patients, other doctors witnessed the same profound effects. Seeing really was believing.

The early data coming in was so impressive, it shifted EyeBio's strategy. It was decided that the company should extend its Series A funding. The original group of venture funds dug deeper into their pockets, and with the addition of Bain Capital Life Sciences, Omega Funds, and Vertex Ventures HC, another $65 million was raised, bringing the total to a cool $130 million (Announced in a press release on 11/14/2023).

AMARONE AMORE

For the twenty-six people with DME and five with wet AMD, in the trial, their typical natural history prognosis was poor. At the back of their eyes were fluid-filled cysts and/or edema, formed by leaky retinal barriers. But with Restoret (EYE103), after a week, four weeks, and finally twelve weeks, in general, many apparently gained visual acuity, and their anatomy, as seen by imaging, returned to near normal in this very early study that would need confirmation by other trials.

These results of the AMARONE trial were presented in February 2024 at the annual Macular Society meeting in Palm Springs, California, by Dr. Charles Wykoff, the director of research at the Retina Consultants of Texas and chairman of the Research and Clinical Trials Committee for Retina Consultants of America. In detail, Wykoff showed that for the

DME patients who received Restoret (EYE103) as a monotherapy, after twelve weeks, they gained on average 11.2 letters on the eye chart, and their central subfield thickness (CST), a measurement of the depth of the central part of the retina, saw excess thickness reduced by 80 percent. All doses—0.15 mg, 0.48 mg, and 0.80 mg—were effective. In the case of the five wet AMD patients who received Restoret (EYE103) in combination with Eylea, Wyckoff revealed after twelve weeks they added 6.8 letters on average, and, even more impressively, their excess CST thickness diminished 100 percent. Again, all the doses—0.05 mg, 0.48 mg, and 0.80 mg—appeared to work in this preliminary study. While two Phase 3 trials of longer duration will be necessary to confirm the safety and efficacy of the drug, as well as for approval, the early data was quite compelling.

In a follow-up interview with the publication *Retinal Physician*, Wykoff said, "This is one of the most interesting early-phase data sets I have ever seen." He went on to comment, "These results are fascinating. We have looked at a lot of other pathways—PDGF (platelet-derived growth factor), kallikrein biology, and integrins, to name just three—but we have never seen another pathway that has such a dramatic benefit beyond VEGF inhibition." Again, only proper randomized controlled clinical trials can accurately prove the efficacy and safety of a drug.

On May 5, 2024, Merck & Co., Inc. (Rahway, New Jersey, USA), known outside the US and Canada as MSD, announced its intention to acquire EyeBio. The company's press release that day stated it would "acquire EyeBio for a $1.3 billion upfront payment and up to $1.7 billion in future milestone payments for a potential value of $3 billion." This had already been unanimously approved by EyeBio's board. Bruce Peacock did a great job leading the EyeBio deal team.

EyeBio's point of view was explained by Kate: "This agreement reflects the hard work of the talented EyeBio team, led by Dr. Guyer, who through this agreement have placed Restoret (EYE103) on a defined development path to patients."

Additionally, Tony and David would bring more to the pharmaceutical giant than just the two molecules in development, they would help "expand the company's presence in ophthalmology." Specifically, the release stated, "The EyeBio team and leadership including founders Dr. David Guyer and Dr. Tony Adamis will leverage their experience and world-class expertise as part of the company to continue their pioneering work to advance the clinical development of Restoret (EYE103) and other ongoing development programs." (From the company's press release of 5/5/2024)

The acquisition was completed on July 11, 2024. EyeBio officially became a "wholly-owned subsidiary" of the company. Exactly a year to the day after Astellas finalized its purchase of Iveric.

THE NEXT PHASE

These corporate machinations did not slow down the development of Restoret (EYE103)—now called MK-3000—in the least. Less than two months after finalizing the acquisition, the company issued a press release heralding the "Initiation of a Phase 2b/3 Clinical Trial for Restoret (EYE103) for the Treatment of Diabetic Macular Edema." (From the company's press release of 9/4/2024)

In keeping with the sentiment of the earlier trial, this one was named, BRUNELLO, after an illustrious Italian red wine, known for its bold character and exceptional aging quality. David was quoted in the release saying this new "trial marks an important milestone as we work with our new colleagues at the company, driven by the common purpose to deliver new, much needed options for patients with diabetic macular edema."

The BRUNELLO trial was designed as "a randomized double-masked Phase 2b/3 trial evaluating the efficacy and safety of two dose levels of intravitreal (IVT) MK-3000 [Restoret (EYE103)] versus active control ranibizumab (Lucentis) in patients with DME." In the first year of the trial, the press release explains, "patients will be randomized 1:1:1 to receive low and high doses of MK-3000 or ranibizumab every four weeks."

Then, “In the second year, the frequency of treatment for participants will shift based on a personalized treatment algorithm.” The goals are to understand the “safety and mean change in best-correct visual acuity from baseline to week 52 in the study eye of the participants.”

According to the press release, “DME impacts an estimated 750,000 people in the United States” and the “prevalence of DME is anticipated to rise with the increasing incidence of diabetes.” As David sees it, “You’ve got to be in ophthalmology if you’re a large pharmaceutical company. Older people, diabetics and obesity are on the rise. Retinal diseases cross these territories. Reflecting on EyeBio’s status as a wholly-owned subsidiary of Merck & Co., Inc. (Rahway, New Jersey, USA), David says, “It’s the best of both worlds. The resources and breadth of the traditional pharmaceutical industry with the speed of biotech. The stars all aligned.”

Chapter 12

MEASURING SUCCESS

AN EYEFUL OF CHANGE

In life, success depends on being in the right place at the right time. That's a given. But it's what you do at that moment that drives the outcome. If Tony took a much-needed nap during Judah Folkman's lecture at Harvard all those years ago, who knows, maybe we'd still be waiting for angiogenesis to be the focus of ocular disease research. Instead, Tony decided to change the trajectory of his career. And talk to David over some linguini.

After originally seeking Genentech's anti-VEGF molecule and being turned away, David may have told himself, "Well, these Big Pharma folks know what they're saying. There's no market for this. And who really wants to be injected in their eye?" And when Marty flew to New York to ask David to form a company, he could have responded, "No, thanks. I'll keep my head down and teach at NYU for the next forty years. It's a sweet gig." Even though Samir knew some of his relatives' pockets were lined with cash, he could easily have felt that raising $8 million from friends and family was too big an ask. While Tony, David, and Samir unquestionably knew they were doing the right thing, it's only in hindsight that the momentousness of their decisions can be appreciated. What's equally important to making those decisions is being in a position where decisions taken are effective. Much of this is chance. Being in the right place at the right time. Yet, luck alone is not enough. It's vital to be prepared and aware, so that when luck strikes, you are ready to act.

Millions and millions of people who would otherwise have gone blind can now see. The treatment of diseases at the back of the eye has been revolutionized. For the most common causes of blindness in the Western world—age-related macular degeneration and diabetic retinopathy—90 percent of patients don't lose vision. The effect of anti-VEGF therapies was immediate. In countries ranging from Scotland to Israel, the number of legally blind people in 2012, eight years after Macugen's FDA approval, was less than half of the tally in 2000.

In the US, intravitreal injections are now the number one billed procedure in all of Medicare for any subspecialty—the market for anti-VEGF therapies is at least $15 billion annually. So much for no one wanting to be injected in their eye! No doubt, penny-pinchers will quibble about the government footing the cost, but imagine what our society would be like if, as life expectancy and obesity increased, so did the hordes of old and overweight blind people. How would that impact everyone's quality of life? Assuming you maintained your health, who would you be taking care of right now or in a few years? Ushering them about their daily activities—everything from driving them to and fro to slicing their vegetables. What effect would that have on your productivity and well-being? Then multiply that by a couple of million. Jon Prenner sees it as a "boiling the frog slowly" scenario: "The development of retinal pharmacologics made an incredible public health improvement that you haven't noticed because our inventions have gotten so much better; our delivery has gotten better as the incidence rate has gone up." He feels that if we had continued on a straight trajectory since 1999, without the invention of anti-VEGF drugs, "it would have been a total wasteland with huge numbers of patients who would have suffered devastating vision loss."

Intravitreal injections have not only become the standard of care for existing therapeutics, but researchers in today's laboratories expect the drugs they are developing will be administered that way when they ultimately journey from the lab bench to the patient's bedside. "The eye is quite a privileged organ," notes Kate Bingham. "If you put [the drug] in the back of the eye, it basically stays put. And so, it gives you flexibility in terms of toxicity because you may have something that, if it was floating around in that concentration, would cause all sorts of side effects in the rest of the body. But because you keep it in the back of the eye, you've got more of a safety check."

Not only has drug delivery been transformed, but each of David's three companies has been built on a different mechanism of action, from anti-VEGF to complement inhibitor and now Wnt agonist. The door is now wide open for researchers to investigate novel approaches. It's easy to imagine that another mode initially explored for an ailment elsewhere in the body winds up applicable in the eye.

Granted, there's still room for improvement. Over time, the effectiveness of treatment diminishes, and there are still large numbers of people whose benefit is suboptimal. This is perhaps why the most significant impact of David's efforts isn't simply measured in patient outcomes to date but lies in opening a whole new paradigm for developing ophthalmic treatments, including the emerging possibilities of combination therapies. Without the dedication of David, Samir, and Tony, and the teams they assembled, it's impossible to say where ophthalmology would be today. They started the dawn of pharmacotherapy for retinal diseases and continue to push the limits today.

FOLLOWING IN THEIR FOOTSTEPS FROM BENCHSIDE TO BEDSIDE

By proving there is a global market for anti-VEGF ophthalmic treatment, to the tune of $15 billion annually with some estimates predicting upwards of $20 billion by 2030, CMOs at Big Pharma companies have eye diseases firmly in their sights—a very different picture from David's first foray at the dawn of the century. The pharmaceutical industry is aware that there are numerous unmet medical needs in ophthalmology, and it is worthwhile exploring eye drug development. Given that the average cost to develop a drug typically falls between $1 billion to $2 billion and that 90 percent of drugs don't get approved, this change of mindset in the industry is a triumph in itself. The reward is worth the risk.

This more open approach to eye diseases by the industry creates an array of opportunities for practicing clinicians. Today, it's far more common to find ophthalmologists filling the roles of chief medical officer, chief scientific officer, or chief development officer at major companies. Considering the minimal training in ophthalmology at medical schools, this is a sign that eye care is finally receiving the attention it warrants. Gone are the days when, as David says, "CMOs didn't know anything about ophthalmology. Most of them didn't even know the names of the diseases. It was completely foreign. They didn't have any interest in going forward."

This evolution has not only broadened the employment landscape for eye doctors, enabling them to have far-reaching influence beyond time-constrained, one-on-one patient care, but it also means that pharma now knows and speaks the language of ophthalmology. Clinical trial designs for eye-related treatments has become less arcane and more pragmatic. Consequently, decision-making is smarter while drug development is more targeted and quicker.

Beyond Big Pharma, there is a legion of smaller companies dedicated to eye disease. Following David's lead, a number of them have been founded or run by ophthalmologists, such as EyePoint, led by Jay Duker, and Ocular Therapeutics, led by Pravin Dugel, both pursuing retinal disease treatments. "The advantage of a biotech is they can move fast; they can be aggressive," says David, "unlike a Big Pharma that might take more time."

Both Duker and Dugel have a background in academia like David and Tony. In the past, relationships between educational institutions and industry were frowned upon. "If you were a consultant back in the 1990s for a drug company, especially as an academic, people looked at you funny," recalls David. "This was a really bad thing. People made me feel guilty, like I was doing something wrong." The perspective has completely reversed. "Today, it seems that almost every chair and professor of ophthalmology at every medical school either has started a company or is associated with a bunch of them." Obviously, it's vital for academics to clearly publicize their industry connections and avoid any conflicts of interest, but David sees tremendous upside to these arrangements: "It's been really important because ophthalmology was always an afterthought for drug treatments." He feels that in the past it was only after developing therapies for other conditions, like cardiovascular illness, that any subsequent use for eye disease was considered: "We got those kind of drugs secondhand, but not usually from primary research."

Interestingly, when David sees academics cross over into pharmaceutical industry vocations, he's observed they, in general, make the transition extremely smoothly. He calls them athletes—academic superstars with exceptional skill sets that can quickly transition to industry. And in Emmett's case, also move into venture capital rapidly and very effectively as well. Talking about these "athletes," he says, "Within six months you would've thought they've been in the industry for twenty-five, thirty years. Part of it is because technically they know everything so well." He feels their professional enthusiasm also plays an important role: "And also it's the energetic level that ophthalmologists have." But he sees that research and development is better suited for this kind of temperament, rather than other pharmaceutical industry areas such as commercialization, manufacturing, or sales.

While academia has proven to be fertile ground for cross-pollination of ophthalmology into pharmaceuticals, David is particularly proud of his own companies acting as breeding grounds for talent. The once professor and chair who taught students and residents at NYU continued to teach as a biotech CEO and trained a new generation. Over twenty alumni of Eyetech and Iveric have become CEOs of their own companies. It marks a profound generational shift—a huge potential to create exciting new treatments has been unleashed.

EYES ON THE PRIZE

Research requires money. Loads of it. Before Eyetech, pharmaceutical interest in eye treatments focused on glaucoma and dry eyes—largely eye drops to lower intraocular pressure or treat redness and similar irritations along with medical devices for doctors to use in their offices. When the greatest return on investment was perceived to be less than $1 billion per year in revenue, eye disease never crossed investors' radar. Changing this perception demanded deep scientific understanding, tremendous foresight, and unrelenting tenacity.

"The idea that you can start and build a biotech company that exclusively pursues eye diseases based on some new elucidation of biology/disease pathophysiology," Srini explicates about all the steps required, "AND that early clinical trials can de-risk the programs, AND that you can ultimately get funded to approval . . . AND that those drugs would be multi-billion-dollar drugs (even while it's a therapy that involves—literally—a needle in your eye). . . Well, I do give a bunch of credit to the three amigos to make that clear to the investment community." He summarizes, "Eyetech especially was eye-opening to both private investors and to Wall Street."

Mike Ross sees another important realization for biotech investors that flows from David's work: Eye doctors are always on the lookout for better therapies. "If you get a drug on the market and people believe it's better, especially in ophthalmology," he asserts, "they're going to use it."

The repercussions of the success of Eyetech and David's subsequent companies have been far reaching. There has been an exponential increase in venture capital funding for ophthalmic biotech start-ups. Additionally, since 2010, billions and billions have been invested in ophthalmological acquisitions and collaborations. Notably, in recent years, there has been a significant rise in investment in innovative therapies including stem cell research and gene therapy, evidence that eye care is at the forefront of scientific inquiry and no longer an afterthought.

However, increased investment doesn't directly improve the odds of finding a particular treatment, and Phase 3 trials remain an incredibly expensive gamble, always a fifty-fifty shot. "Being an investor in biotech is nerve-wracking," states David. "It's definitely not for the faint of heart." However, the numbers game means with more research arriving at this point, more eye treatments will be approved. The bigger the arsenal of drugs available to eye doctors, the greater the choice they will have to address their patients' needs.

Kate explains David's impact on the VC world this way: "The brilliance about David is not just that he came up with multiple fantastic drugs, but those have been new first-in-class drugs, which enables the whole field to develop, which enables patients to get treated better." Macugen is a case in point. There's little doubt that Lucentis wouldn't have been developed so quickly without a precursor, then rapidly followed by other anti-VEGF therapies. As treatment areas mature, devising combination therapies expands the range of options available, allowing doctors to fill in gaps and customize approaches. Treatment won't be one-size-fits-all, and as our understanding of genetics increases, so will the ability to tailor medication to suit individual needs. "Not every patient is going to respond to every drug," says Kate.

Market conditions are fickle. There will always be investment cycles driven by macroeconomic or geopolitical events; plus, sentiments shift, and risk appetites alter with the success or failure of high-profile companies. But the big picture is that ophthalmology isn't relegated anymore to a second-tier status.

In a world increasingly under the sway of visual culture, isn't this the way things should be?

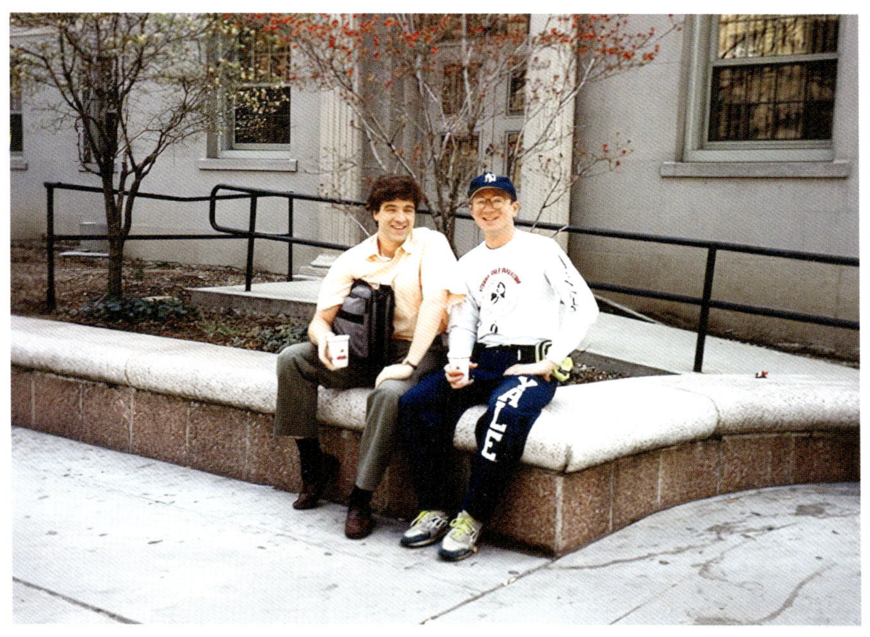

TONY AND DAVID OUTSIDE THE HARVARD LABORATORY

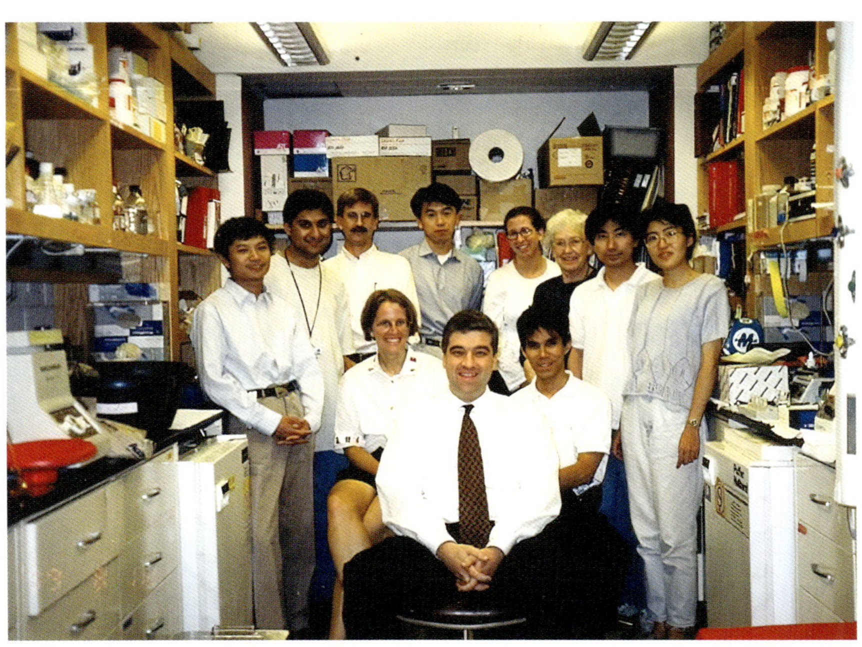

TONY'S LABORATORY

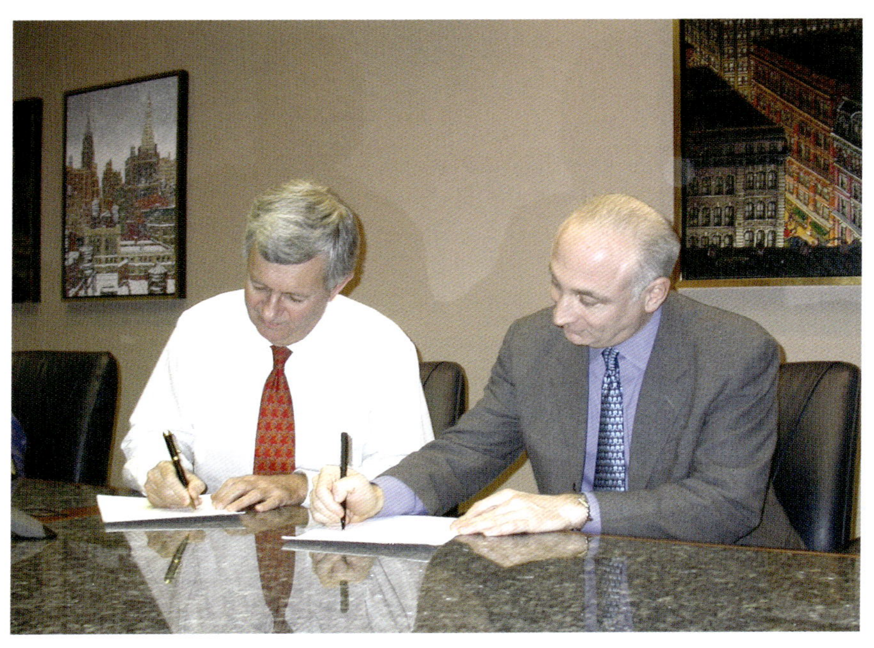

PFIZER AND EYETECH CEOS SIGNING THE DEAL

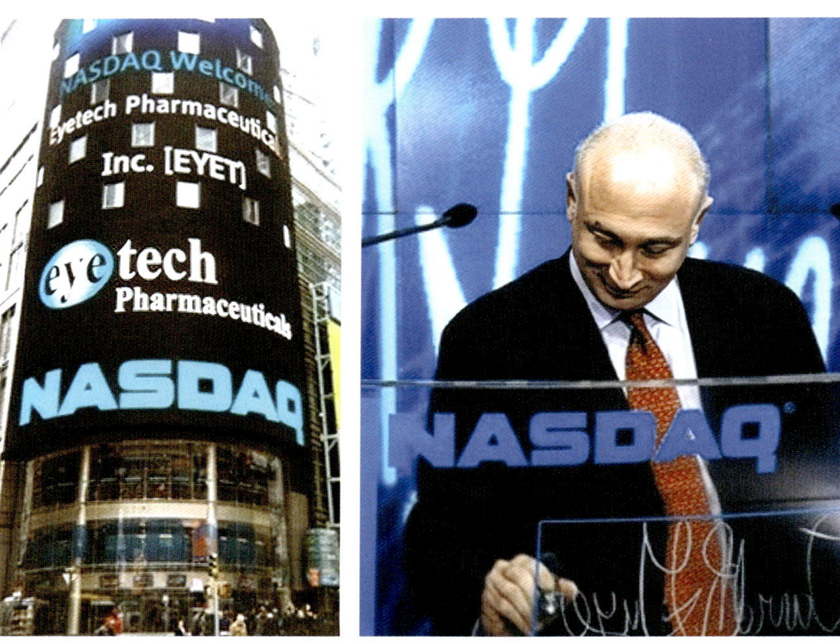

EYETECH GOES PUBLIC ON JANUARY 30, 2004 (LEFT),
DAVID GUYER SIGNING AT NASDAQ (RIGHT)

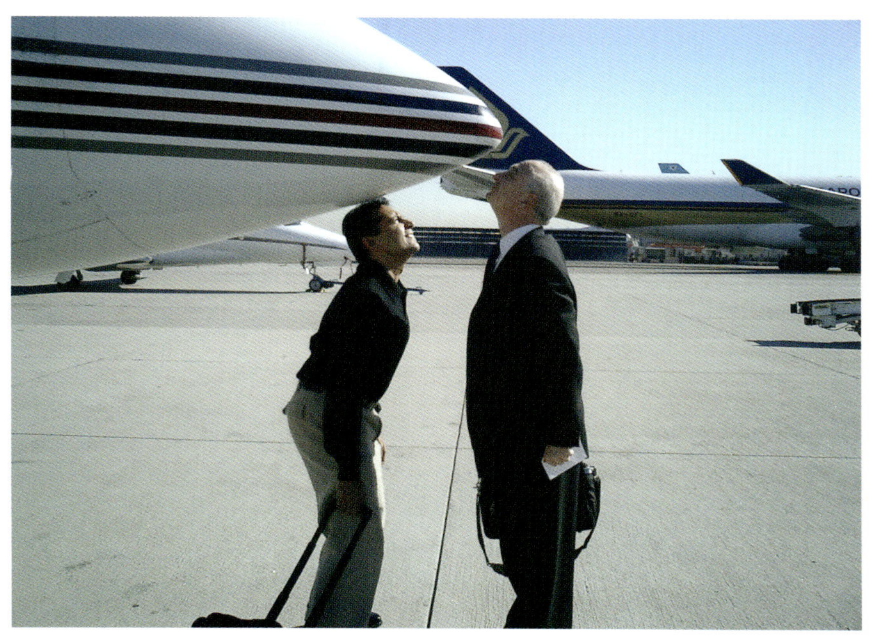

SAMIR AND DAVID

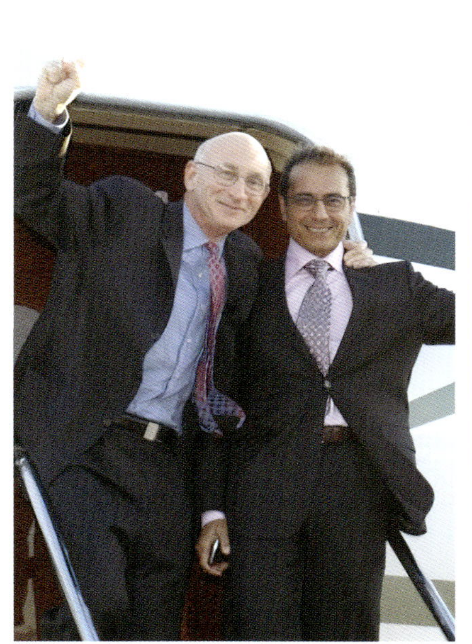

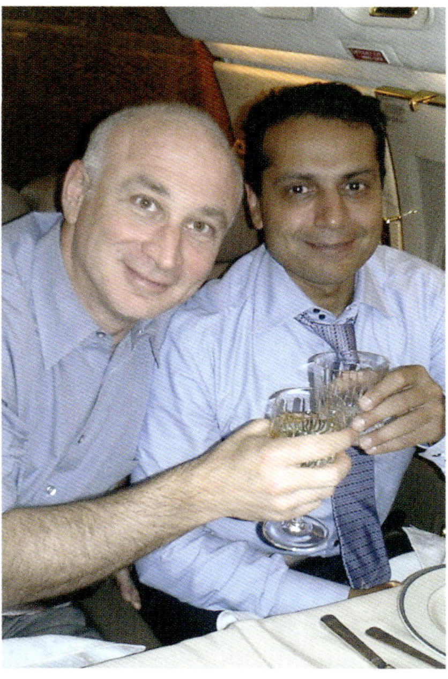

OPHTHOTECH ROADSHOW (LEFT), DAVID AND SAMIR (RIGHT)

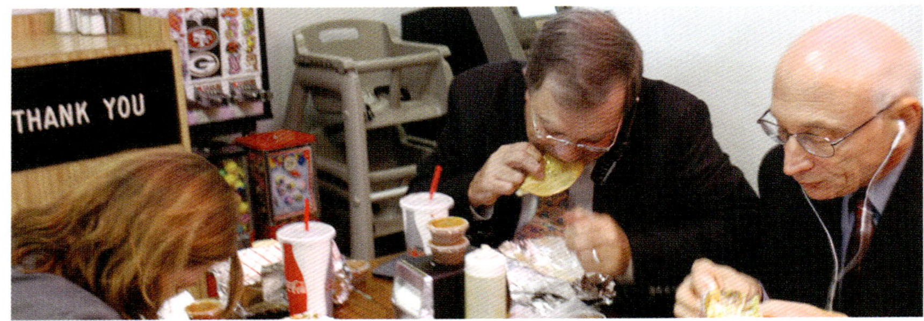

OPHTHOTECH ROADSHOW: SAN FRANCISCO

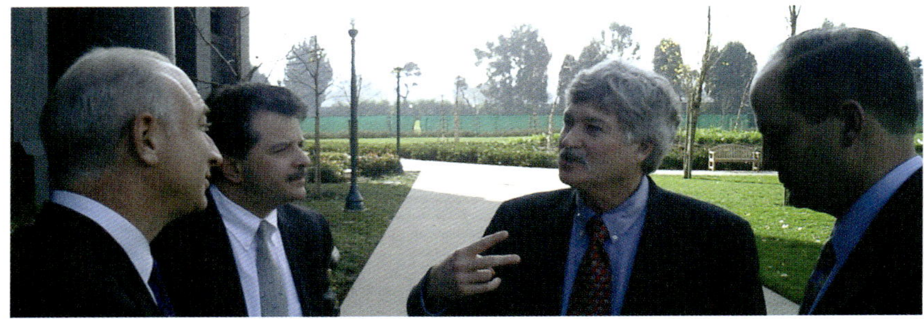

DAVID, GLENN SBLENDORIO, MARTY GLICK, AND PAUL CHANEY

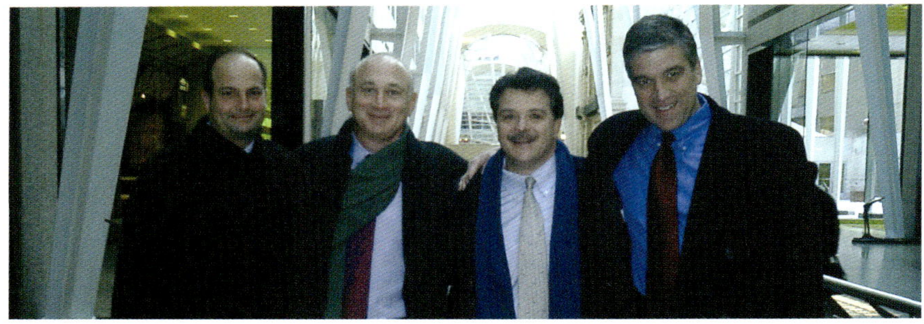

PAUL, DAVID, GLENN, AND TONY

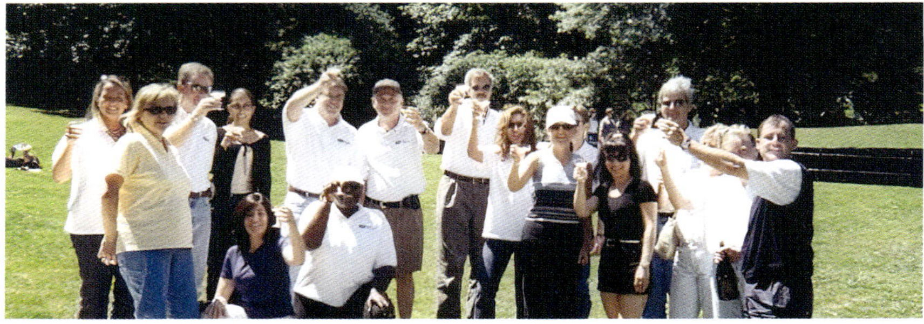

OPHTHOTECH CENTRAL PARK PARTY

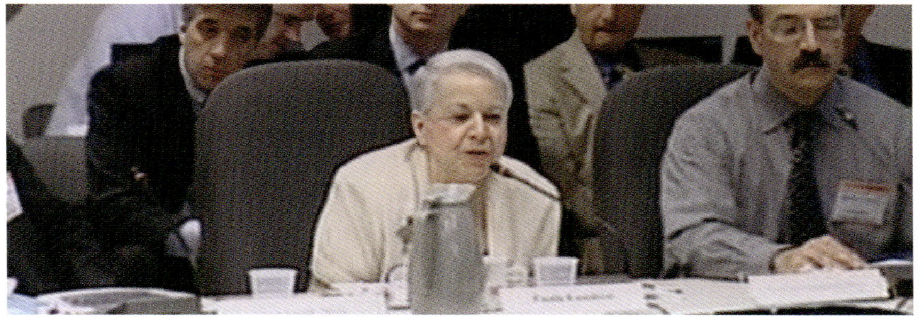

FDA ADVISORY MEETING

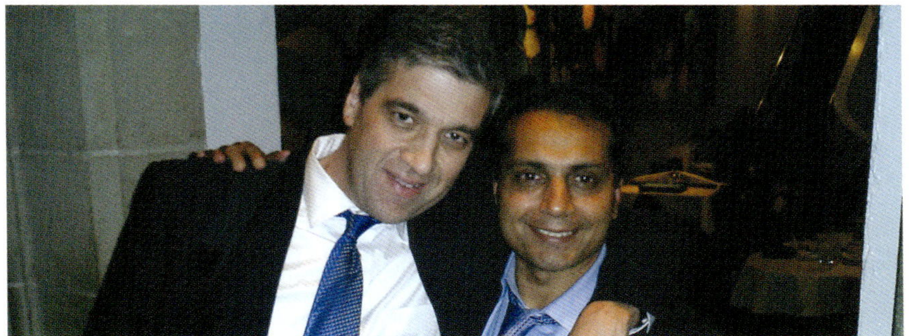

TONY AND SAMIR

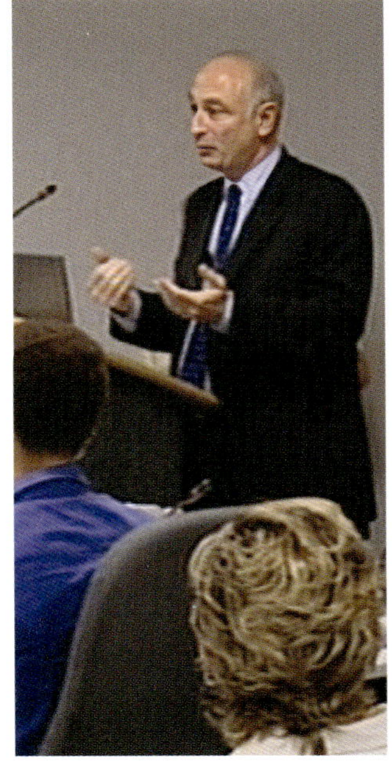

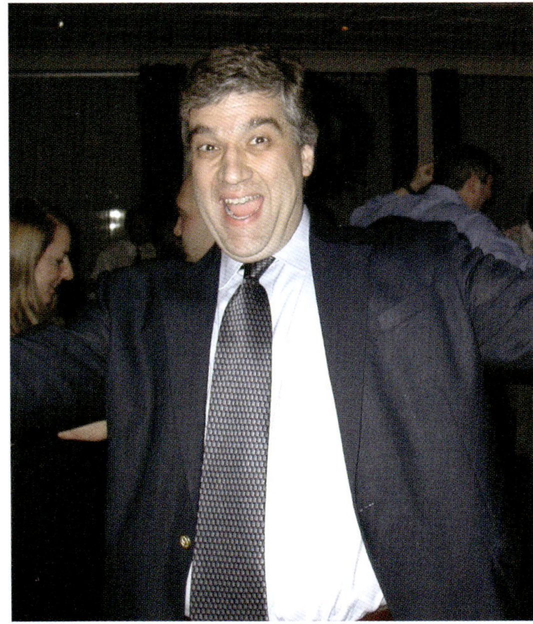

FDA ADVISORY MEETING (LEFT), FDA APPROVAL (RIGHT)

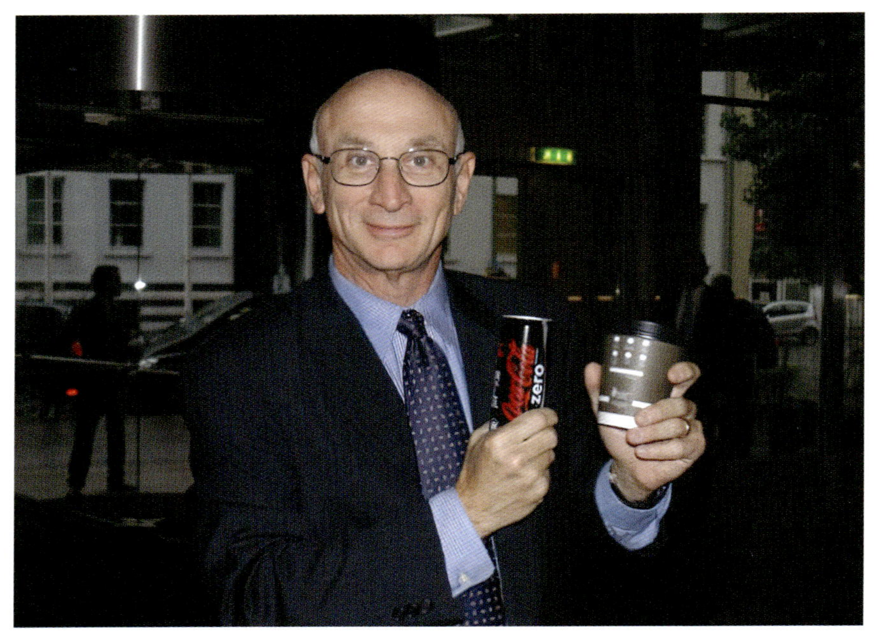

CAFFEINE, CAFFEINE, AND MORE CAFFEINE . . .

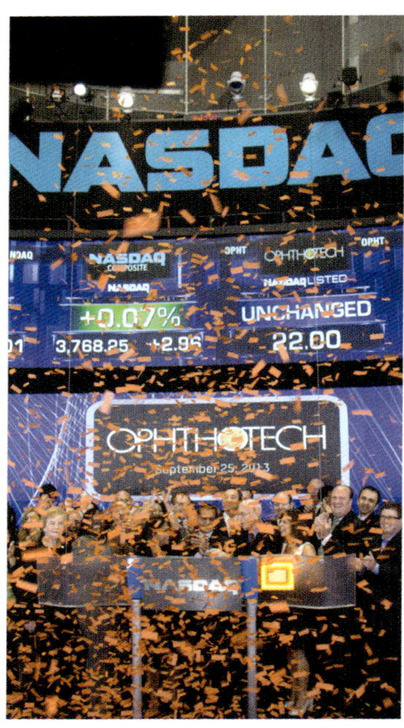

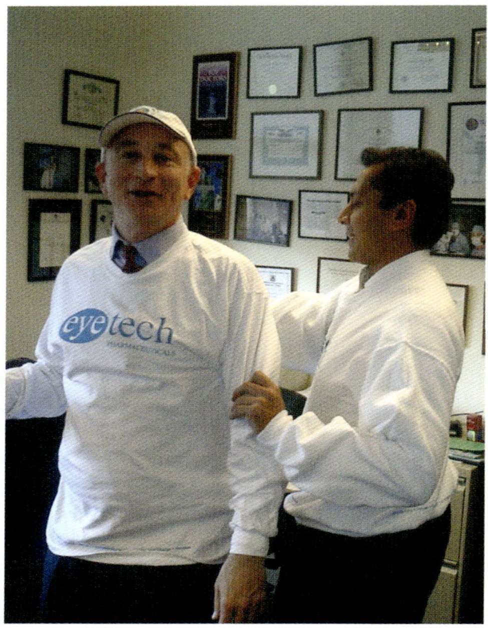

ANOTHER BIG DAY AT THE NASDAQ (LEFT), DAVID AND SAMIR (RIGHT)

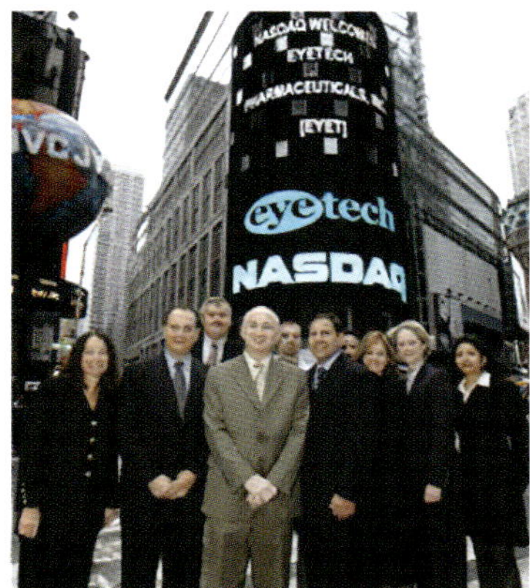

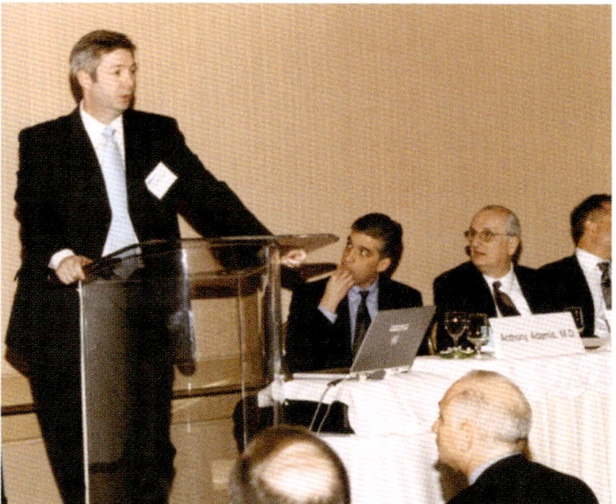

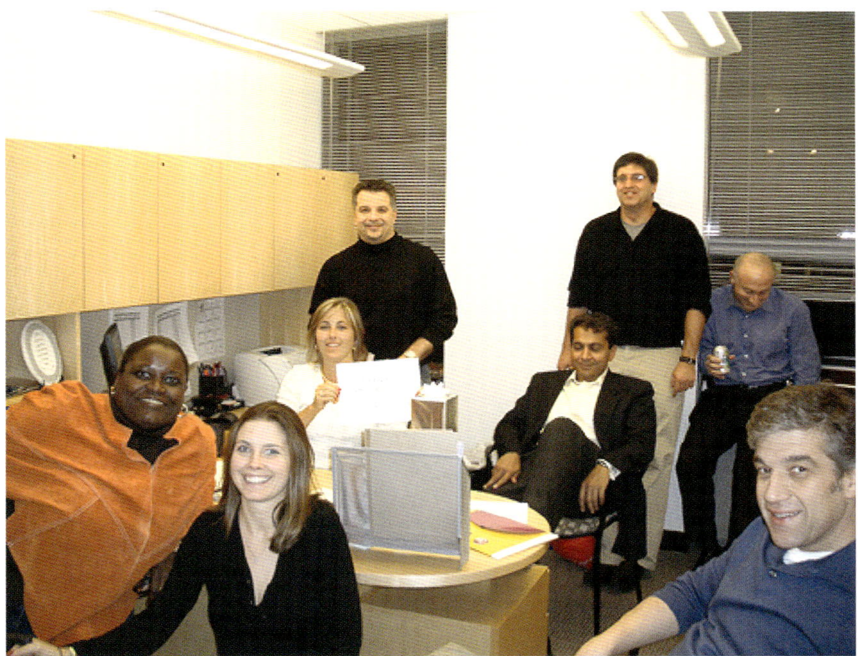

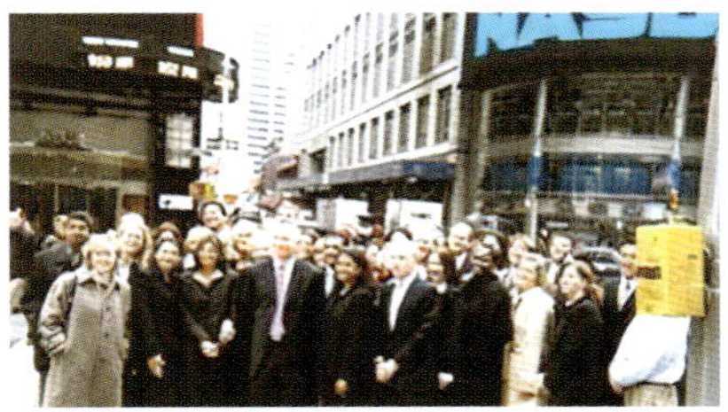

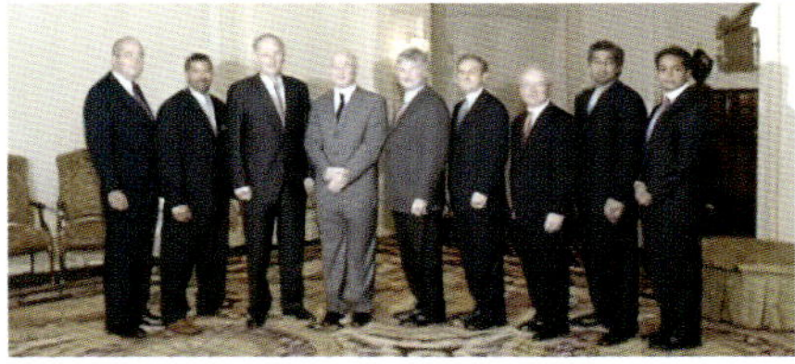

EYETECH BOARD

EYETECH CULTURE—WE WORK HARD . . .

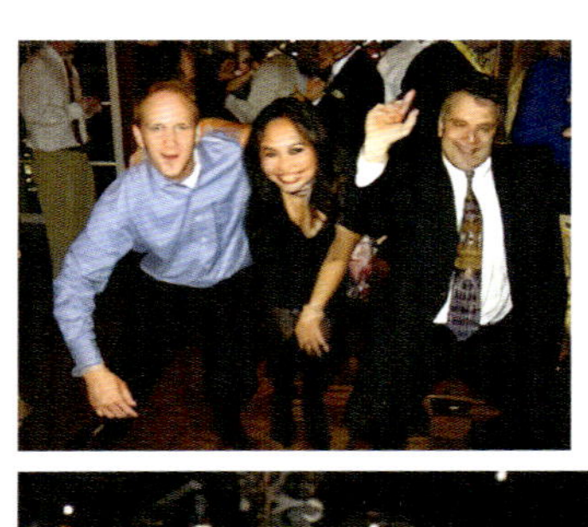
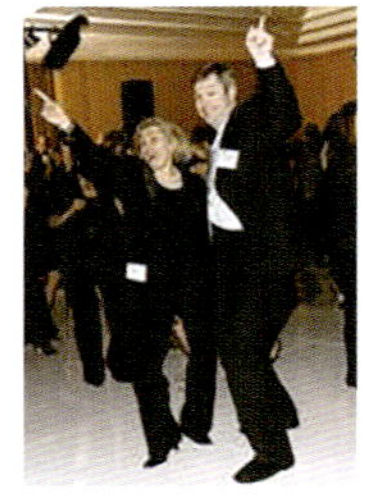
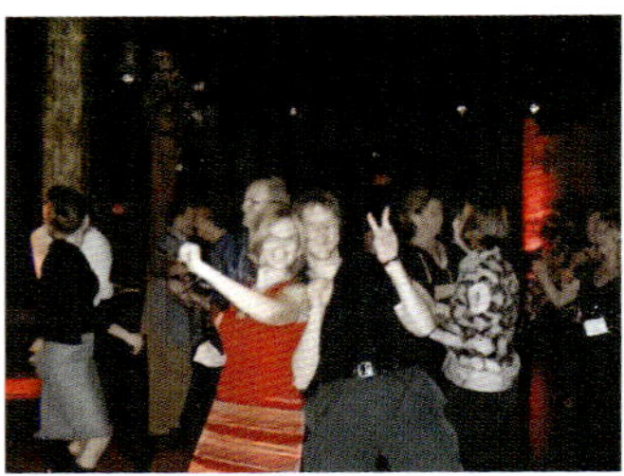
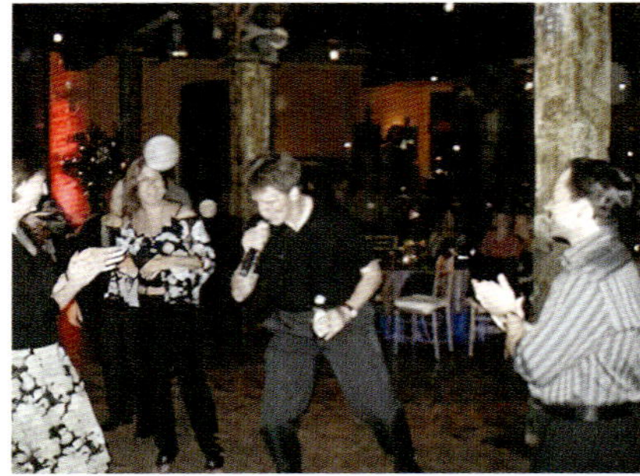
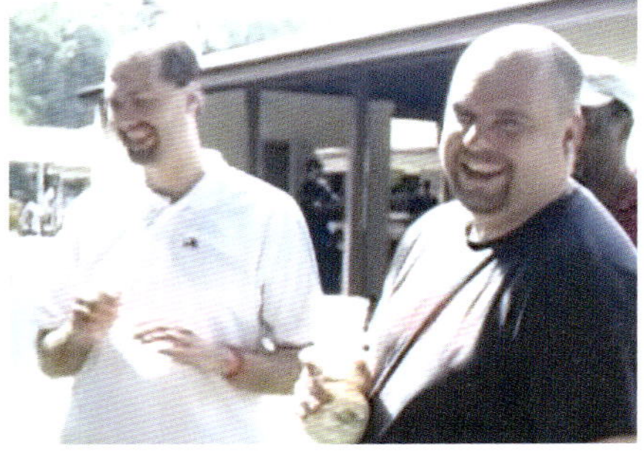
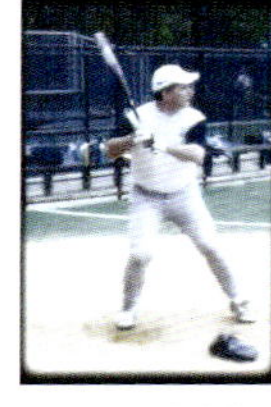
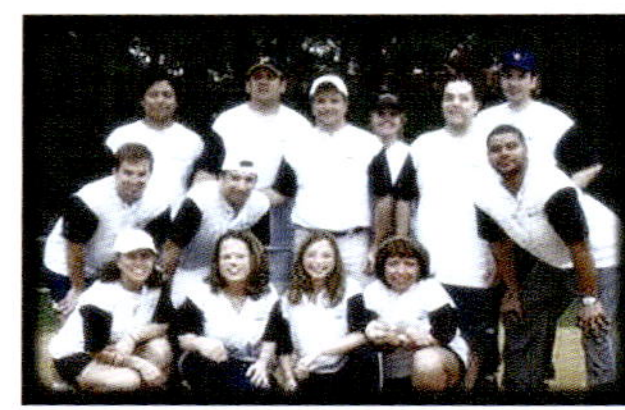
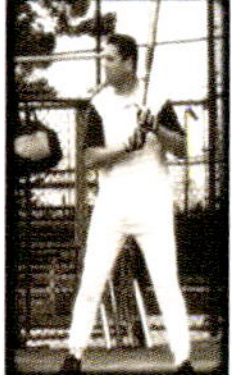
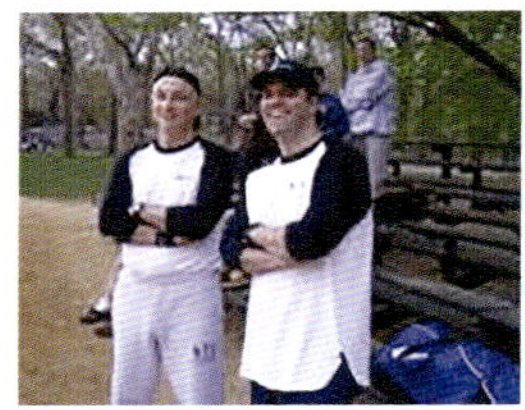
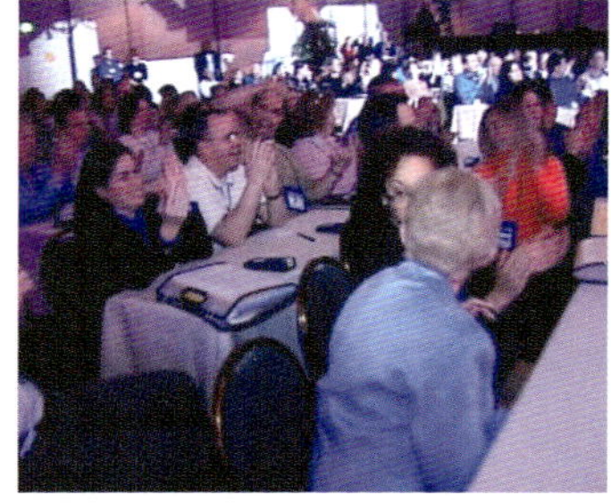
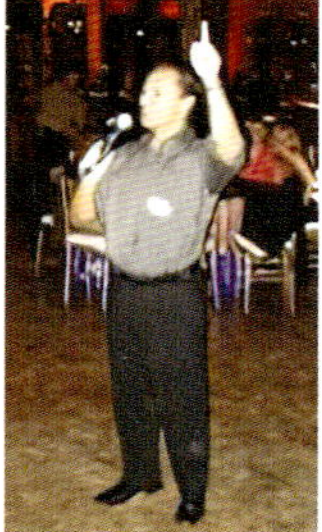
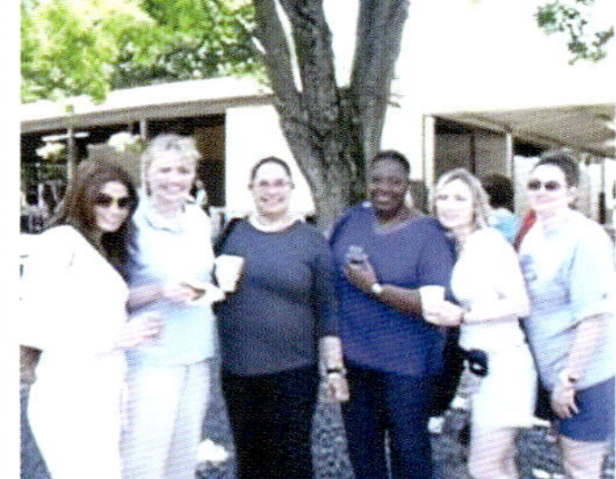
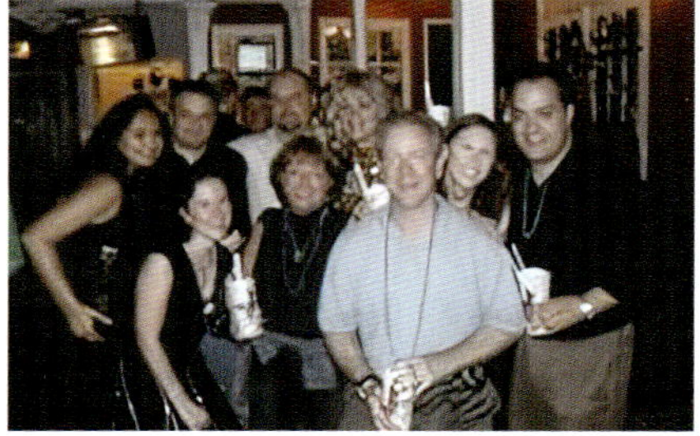
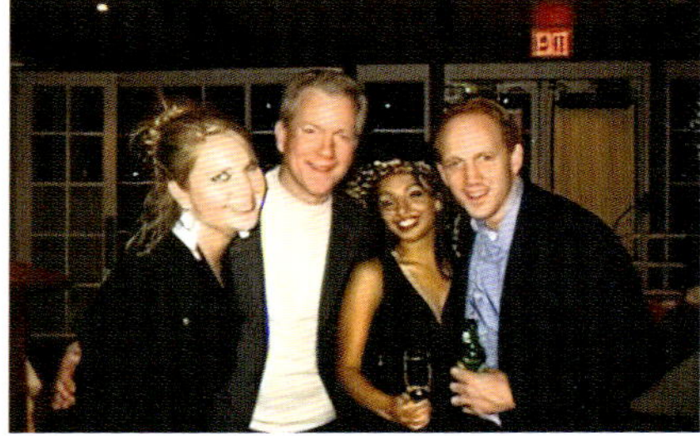

... WE PLAY HARD

EPILOGUE

"We were a bunch of doctors that knew nothing about business or how to run a company," says David in retrospect. "In many ways, I was the least likely person to do this. I was a pure academic. I was the person that you would've predicted to be in academia, writing papers and giving talks forever. Not an entrepreneur. Not a businessperson."

The motivation to change something inherently wrong is very powerful. For David, Tony, and Samir, laser was the orthodoxy that needed to be toppled. It didn't slow vision loss much and was largely useless for the majority of patients. In the early 1990s, through Tony's work with Judah Folkman, an alternative was emerging, but there was no clear pathway from the laboratory to the clinic. It's one thing to publish results in medical journals, another entirely to manufacture, effectively test, and distribute drugs. Especially when you must establish the market first.

What would have happened if Marty hadn't called David after his failure to get Genentech interested in fighting AMD? It's impossible to say. David is certainly tenacious. Perhaps eventually he would have found a way. But Marty's desire to open a back channel and David's willingness to learn the business—trading his professorship for what he calls a "street MBA"—show you must be open to change yourself to broadly effect change. Having plunged headfirst into the deep end, David not only quickly learned to swim but proved to be a champion, three times over. Along the way, David honed his skills and asserts there are lessons learned that apply to business in general, regardless of the industry.

As a venture capitalist, in addition to his experience as CEO, David maintains, "Keeping ego in check is vital." David says, "You can often see successful CEOs are the ones with low egos versus the overly egotistical ones that don't last and fail." Moving down the ladder, he advises leaders to "hire athletes" when building their teams. People with skills, flexibility, endurance, and creativity. In David's case, "it was academic medicine superstars." Micromanagement is unnecessary with individuals like Tony or Emmett Cunningham, who, after serving as SVP of medical strategy at Eyetech, wove together a distinguished career working in a leading teaching hospital while being a serial entrepreneur and top investor, including a stretch as senior managing director at Blackstone's Life Sciences Group. "You hire great people and you delegate," David expounds. "You have daily meetings with teams like a sports coach. You only become a control freak when there's a problem and then you jump in. But otherwise, you just let great, talented people go and do their thing."

As we've seen, David is also willing to embrace people lacking experience but with the intelligence to learn new skills quickly. In these instances, David has replicated the exposure to business he received from Marty and John McLaughlin. Together with the temperament you'd expect from a veteran of academia, he has skillfully passed along the knowledge he's acquired on the job.

When engaging new talent, David looks for some unusual qualities in a person's character. "The best thing," he maintains, "is to hire people who have paranoid and obsessive-compulsive traits." He doesn't suggest bringing on board people who are fully encumbered by these conditions. What is important is that they have a heightened awareness of what's going on around them in the business and the capacity to fully apply themselves when developing solutions. It is important to always look ahead and see what could go wrong, no matter how unlikely, and to have a plan how to handle them should they occur.

The key to it all lies in motivation. Why be in business in the first place? Even though David's enterprises have created $10 billion of value, success for David and all the people involved in his businesses has consistently been measured in patient outcomes, not dollars. Put simply, are they helping people see better? Ultimately, there is nothing more satisfying than giving the gift of sight. Unquestionably the most rewarding aspect of David, Tony, and Samir's transition from academia and clinical practice to the world of therapeutics, is doing this at a global scale.

According to the American Academy of Ophthalmology, the average eye doctor sees about one hundred patients per week, roughly five thousand in a year. For David to individually treat a million patients would take two hundred years. "It's a more satisfying thing," David acknowledges of his efforts, "because the amount of people you can help is absolutely exponential." One way to look at is that in less than a generation, David, Tony, Samir, and their teams have done a few millennia's worth of work. This magnitude is only achievable by working at an industrial scale. David's transition from clinical practice and academia to biotech and venture capital then ultimately to Big Pharma has allowed him to see ophthalmology from several different points of view. On many levels, gaining this multilayered insight is as revolutionary as the drugs he's developed. But like any revolution, it hasn't been without its battles.

A SEAT AT THE TABLE

First, David had to recognize, with the help of an industry insider, Denis, that despite the failure of the interferon trial, building the infrastructure for clinical trials that dealt with back-of-the-eye diseases was, in fact, a victory. Indeed, the very building block of his future. Still, subsequent efforts to partner with Big Pharma were rebuffed, resulting in Eyetech, an independent biotech company. Even then, David understood that Pfizer had to step in to achieve the scale required to go to market with Macugen. Similarly, Izervay landed with Astellas.

The initial resistance was Big Pharma's inability to see the market potential for retinal treatments. But there was a flip side to this lack of vision, one that affected David on a much more personal level. Inside ophthalmology, the medical establishment reacted to David's embrace of the pharma industry with some disdain. "In the beginning," states David "there was criticism from other retinal docs, saying 'How dare you work for industry, or even consult!'" This led to David questioning his intentions: "Am I doing something evil here working with industry?"

It's possible that a few factors influenced this regrettable behavior. Change is tough. Human nature is to resist it, particularly as you get older. And if your status has been built on something with shaky foundations, then adopting a defensive posture can quickly turn aggressive. But there's likely more to it than just kneejerk reflexiveness. The type of success David and others have been party to in biotech often leads to envy. While David has been slower to pick up on this, others have witnessed it in action. Jon puts his finger on it: "He has been so successful, while being so generous, that people get pretty jealous." Of all our emotions, jealousy is the root of our least becoming and most irrational impulses.

Jealousy also blinds us. When you resentfully focus on someone's success, it's easy to overlook the struggles they endured to get there. Macugen was a triumph of initiative and timing. The race to beat Genentech resulted from the biotech giant's own early myopia—witnessed firsthand by David. The sale to OSI was fortuitous in many ways, and the advent of Lucentis (albeit self-cannibalized by Avastin) rapidly exposed all false assumptions about Macugen's future market share, making the Eyetech team appear doubly lucky. In the wake of this drama, how easy is it to diminish the achievement of being the first to put anti-VEGF treatments in patients' eyes?

If the Eyetech team had any residual cockiness, their experience during the Ophthotech years with Fovista surely dashed it. The failure of the drug led to the hardest times for both David and Samir. "We couldn't have been more down," reflects David. "Many people were upset and shocked."

"And then, of course, when Iveric was sold for six billion, all of a sudden we were gigantic heroes again." David reflects, "It shows the lack of sophistication and reasonability of people. Through their eyes, they don't get it." The fickleness of humans can be disheartening. In the end, it makes David appreciate individuals who think for themselves and understand what's really at stake.

TABLES TURNED

For David, the ultimate vindication doesn't come from Iveric being the biggest sale ever in ophthalmic biotech but instead from surveying today's ophthalmological landscape and seeing the happy marriage of academia and industry. A generational change has followed in his footsteps. "Now, so many years later," he says with uncharacteristic pride, "every academic, even virtually every chairperson of an eye department is involved with founding a company or is chief medical officer, or consultant, or whatever for this company or that company." Not only does this show how seriously eye disease is now taken but that there exists a deep understanding that it takes tremendous resources to turn theory into reality.

It's no longer enough to earn respectability with a good idea; putting it into action is what counts.

The flowering of ophthalmic biotech companies since the appearance of Eyetech is not only due to its financial success but also because David has tilled the soil of future ventures—literally as a biotech operator but also as a mentor. David, in his acceptance speech, receiving the Harvard Medical School Department of Ophthalmology 2024 Distinguished Innovator Award, noted, "One of the things I'm most proud of is that over twenty people who have worked in my companies have gone on to become CEOs of their own companies. Getting that next generation of people to lead companies has been really, really exciting." It's a feeling that brings him back to his origins as a teacher to numerous medical students, residents, and fellows when he was a professor.

BELIEVING IS SEEING

The most important advice David imparts is "you've got to believe in yourself and take chances." It sounds simple, but it takes immense confidence. There is nothing benign about unseating orthodoxy. He reflects on his experience with intravitreal injections: "Everybody told us you couldn't do it, but we thought we could. We could have very easily been influenced by the majority. But we had such conviction." He sees the same principle behind his involvement with the pharmaceutical industry: "The only way these drugs would get approved was with their help."

"Do what you believe in and don't get swayed by people who are telling you something that doesn't feel right to you. That's the big thing," David summarizes. "Whether it be intravitreal injections, or the professor that told me that I was wasting my time with research on drug treatments for retinal diseases, I could have very easily listened to the establishment, and we wouldn't be here. So, you have to believe in what you think is right and go for it. Or you never make any change."

This philosophy has brought us multiple different mechanisms to fight blindness at the back of the eye. Is there more to come? Time will tell. For now, David and his team are excited to be embraced by Big Pharma.

Ironically, for someone who escaped academics, David describes his new work life in Big Pharma as educational and invigorating: "I'm learning a lot. I did academia. I did VC. I did small biotech. I'm now learning Big Pharma while leading EyeBio, as a subsidiary, and it's fascinating. I'm enjoying this experience." For a man who perennially operates at top speed, he isn't troubled. "There are so many positives at Big Pharma, that I'm finding it fascinating." Taking on a new challenge is appealing to David: "I always keep telling people I had three careers. Well, now I feel like I've had four."

Contemporary success is defined by Silicon Valley. It's easy to grasp how a novel computer code can be infinitely replicated and deployed instantly around the planet. We're accustomed to digital platforms producing wealth from scale. In a world habituated to digital disruption, it's hard to recognize the far-reaching effect of something biological and administered by humans, even if the technology and science behind the creation and manufacturing of its medicinal molecules are revolutionary.

But next time you gaze at your phone and its floating sea of apps, remind yourself that for any of its wizardry to have value, you need to be able to see it. When not going blind is something we can all take for granted, that is the ultimate success.

THE END

IAN'S NOTE

When your father is an ophthalmologist, you grow up thinking, "This is what all doctors are like." Part of the fun of writing this book was discovering what outliers in the medical professional eye doctors really are. Eyeballs are for oddballs.

My father, Dr. Theo Keldoulis, retired from clinical practice in 1999, just before the founding of Eyetech. It's been "eye opening" to learn what happened next in ophthalmology. Although he operated frequently on patients' eyes for all kinds of conditions, I doubt my father ever administered an intravitreal injection, certainly not for retinal diseases.

What he did do was start the Gift of Sight Society to fund ophthalmic research in Australia (the society eventually morphed into Australian Vision Research). As president of the Royal Australian and New Zealand College of Ophthalmology he was convinced of the value of ongoing exploration of medical possibilities. Learning about the complexity, risk, and perseverance required to go from "lab bench to bedside" has been utterly fascinating to me.

While the money at stake in this process is mind blowing, one thing that has consistently stuck me is that money is never the motivating force. Without exception everyone in this book finds the greatest satisfaction in helping patients see better.

This rings true to me. My father always said, if he had his life over again, he'd do exactly the same thing—with the possible change of specializing in pediatric ophthalmology, because he felt that helping children had even greater impact. As I approach the latter years of my life, I'm very grateful Dr. Guyer and his companions have paid attention to a disease affecting the elderly.

I used to joke with my father that he gave people sight, while I gave them something to look at. I hope you enjoy reading this book as much as I have writing it.

—IAN KELDOULIS

ACKNOWLEDGMENTS

Bringing to light the multi-decade story of *Unblinded* was the result of a tremendous amount of memory recall and research. This could only have happened with the insights, contributions, and collective memory of a multitude of people.

This long journey would never have begun without Tony Adamis and Samir Patel. We are incredibly grateful to Tony and Samir for their steadfast commitment to improving ophthalmic therapeutics over the years, their devoted, amazing friendships as well as their assistance crafting this story of which they are main characters. Thanks so much to Marty Glick and the late John McLaughlin who were great mentors as well as fantastic "out-of-the box" thinkers. Eyetech simply wouldn't have happened without them.

Special thanks must be given to Katherine Burke and Evelyn Harrison, whose tag-team recounting of events that provided the narrative spine of the book was equally informative and entertaining. Gratitude is also due to their colleagues who took the time to impart their experiences, wisdom, and colorful stories, including Glenn Sblendorio, Bruce Peacock, Lillian Vazquez, Harsha Murthy, Denis O'Shaughnessy, and Loni da Silva. We are especially grateful to Sarah Milsom, who on top of her great work as COO at EyeBio took on the responsibility of shepherding this book through its final stages of development. And from beginning to end David's executive assistant, Mala Hintzen, director, corporate administration, has always been a very essential and incredible worker at all three start-ups, using her miraculous powers to bend time and create holes in David's schedule as well as filling crucial gaps in knowledge all while maintaining a very positive outlook. She always makes David even more efficient.

Of course, science is the foundation of the revolution captured in these pages, and credit must be awarded to the cadre of scientists whose interest and enthusiasm have propelled David, Tony, and Samir forward and rendered the intricate workings of retinal therapeutics understandable. In particular, we appreciate the thoughtful sharing of knowledge by the late Judah Folkman at Harvard Medical School. Also, at Harvard, Joan Miller's singular contributions have greatly advanced our understanding of anti-VEGF therapies along with Patricia D'Amore, Eric Ng, Lloyd Paul Aiello, and the late Dave Shima. And if it weren't for Evangelos Gragoudas, Donald D'Amico, and others taking David as a retinal fellow at Harvard, this incredible story may never have happened. Napoleone Ferrara's endeavors at Genentech are a key component of the science behind the treatments at the heart of this book, and "Napo" deserves our deepest gratitude. Also, George Yancopolous and Len Schleifer of Regeneron need to be singled out for thanks. At the other side of the planet, Andrew Cuthbertson graciously provided insight into the mechanisms of anti-VEGF therapies and the original challenges of bringing them to ophthalmology. Thanks are also due to David Antonetti, Sang Han, Jeremy Nathans, and Sekar Seshagiri. Ultimately, the development of treatments for retinal disease would have stalled had not the two key executives at the head of Gilead, the late John Martin and John Milligan, understood that David's team was best suited to unlock the potential of their company's molecule.

It's vital to acknowledge David's early college mentorship by the late J. P. Trinkaus, a professor at Yale who first sparked David's interest in research, and also the late Dick Green, Stuart Fine, and Neil Miller, who convinced David to go into ophthalmology as a medical student at Johns Hopkins. At Johns Hopkins' Wilmer Eye Institute, David was grateful for the camaraderie of his fellow residents Lloyd Paul Aiello, Bob Avery, Dean Eliott, Tamara Fountain, Mami Iwamoto, Paul Lee, Pedro Lopez, Al

Maguire, Robert Maloney, Peter McDonnell, Sumit Nanda, Terry O'Brien, Arun Patel, Dan Schwartz, Bill Smiddy, Jon Talamo, Marco Zarbin, and, indeed, all the other basement dwellers. While at Manhattan Eye and Ear, David is thankful to have had Jack Dodick as his chair and mentor. David also appreciates all the deans and professors at NYU whom he worked alongside. We would also like to thank all the key opinion leaders and principal investigators who've helped shape the course of retinal treatments over the past few decades, especially Bob Avery, Francesco Bandello, Kristine Baumane, Rubens Belfort, Alan Bird, Mark Blumenkranz, David Boyer, Neil Bressler, Susan Bressler, Dave Brown, Sandy Brucker, Peter Campochiaro, Usha Chakraborty, Antonio Ciardella, the late Gabriel Coscas, Karl Csaky, Don D'Amico, François Devin, Pravin Dugel, Jay Duker, Chiara Eandi, Michel Eid Farah, Yale Fisher, Bailey Freund, Tom Friberg, the late Wayne Fung, Kurt Gitter, Evangelos Gragoudas, Victor Gonzalez, Julia Haller, Larry Halperin, Jeff Heier, Allen Ho, Glenn Jaffe, Michael Jumper, Barry Kuppermann, Guna Laganovska, Dan Martin, Jordi Mones, Aaron Naigel, Eric Nudleman, Carmen Puliafito, Maddalena Quaranta, Carl Regillo, Elias Reichel, Federico Ricci, Francisco Rodriguez, Phil Rosenfeld, Reggie Sanders, Andrew Schachat, Howard Schatz, Patricio Schlottmann, Steve Schwartz, Larry Singerman, Rishi Singh, Jason Slakter, John Sorenson, Giselle Soubrane, Eric Souied, Rick Spaide, Giovanni Staurenghi, George Williams, Charles Wykoff, Marco Zarbin, plus so many others! Beyond the world of retina specialists, David treasures his friendship with fellow New York ophthalmologists Jay Wisnicki and Harry Koster and Boston ophthalmologist Jon Talamo.

David's education was greatly enhanced by the ophthalmological luminary Larry Yannuzzi, who imbued with his love of medicine, taught David about the retina, and early on supported his research and worldwide lecturing. Larry was instrumental in teaching David about the macula, clinical research and how to present at meetings. David's chair at Wilmer, Mort Goldberg, shaped David's understanding of academic medicine, administration, and a love of research, teaching him the 5 P's: "proper planning prevents poor performance." In turn, the medicines David, Tony and Samir have introduced to patients have been carefully developed and stewarded by the rigorous and creative work of Emmett Cunningham, Kourous Rezaei, Matt Feinsod, Keith Baker, Charles Miller, and Daniel Janer. Special thanks to Jon Prenner for the great work he has done as EyeBio CMO and for his fantastic friendship. And thanks again to Emmett, who David has known longer than anyone else mentioned in this book, for constantly encouraging him to write this story.

This book attests to the difficulties and expense of going from lab bench to bedside. Without investors who cannot only analyze the risks but are willing to take them, no groundbreaking new medicines would ever materialize. It's imperative to thank the Patel investor group, led by Dr. S. M. Patel, for providing our first funding. Thankfully, Hingge Hsu opened the door to SV Health Investors, and it has never closed. SV, led originally by the late Henry Simon, then under the stewardship of Jim Garvey, has been both an audacious stakeholder and a safe haven. Both leaders have been great mentors to David. We are grateful this ongoing relationship continues under the guidance of Kate Bingham, Mike Ross, and Alex Badamchi-Zadeh. David has loved working closely with Mike, and especially wants to thank Kate for her confidence in him and her great wisdom. Thanks are also due to Damion Wicker and Srini Akkaraju. Srini was not only prescient about the opportunity for retinal therapeutics but provided understanding of the venture capitalist perspective on investing in the sector. Srini's engagement was evinced as a board member for both Eyetech and EyeBio. We are also grateful to Tom Elden and his family office, Robert Glassman (when at Merrill Lynch) and Kurt Wheeler, who helped us when at MPM. Venture capital contributions and great advice from Mitchell Blutt, Christine Brennan, Olga Danilchanka, Bernard Davitian, Peter Dudek, Thomas Dyrberg, Len Finer, Nicholas Galakatos, Lutz Giebel, Jack Kenney, Adam Koppel, Ed Penhoet, Otello Stampacchia, Rafaele Tordjman, Andreas Wallnoefer, Amir Zamani, and others, have also been essential to our success, and we are highly appreciative of their efforts, as well as our bankers Mike

Gaito, Tony Gibney, Mark Robinson, Marshall Smith, Steve Harr, and others, who helped get the financial ball rolling. Thanks are also due to Eric Tokat and the Centerview team, as well as Mark Robinson, Alan Hartman, and Ivan Farman and the BOA team.

Once seeded, the businesses in this book have blossomed due to individuals whose management skills are combined with scientific and financial expertise. At Eyetech, Paul Chaney brought his enthusiasm and experience from Pharmacia to steer the young company's operations. Thanks also to David Hallal and his incomparable sales force. Evelyn Harrison, Loni da Silva, and Glenn Sblendorio together conveyed over a third of a century of hard won knowledge in pharma to the fledgling company. They repeated this at Ophthotech, where Bruce Peacock also came onboard after decades dealing with the business side of biotech, and he deserves special thanks for his great work at EyeBio as well.

All three companies have excelled under exemplary executive and developmental leadership. We thank Douglas Altschuler, Todd Anderman, Michael Atieh, Rocco Auletta, Walesca Ayala, Kevin Berth, Desiree Beutelspacher, Steve Bettis, Frances Betts, Tom Biancardi, Henric Bjarke, Doug Brooks, Harry Brown, Leslie Bucker, Stu Builder, Pat Carpenter, David Carroll, Anthony Castiglia, Tamiko Comeaux, Sonia Cruz, Tom Ciulla, Mike Davies, Jon Dines, the late Richard Everett, Matt Feinsod, Laura Fougman, Beth Fucito, Kathy Galante, Carrie Gallagher, Colin Goddard, Mauro Goldbaum, Matt Haughey, Jill Healy, Patrick Healy, Karin Hehenberger, Erin Henry, Nabila Hoque, Forbes Huang, Martin Johansson, Patricia Johnson, Barrett Katz, Doug Kollmorgen, the late Doug Kornbrust, Laura Kupsch, Karen Langenberg, Divya Manek, Sheri Manson, Harvey Masonson, David Millband, Bryce Miller, Marlene Modi, Jeff Nau, Andrew Piringer, Tim Piringer, Mike Rafa, Nancy Ramirez, Vera Reinstadler, Melanie Rice, David Robinson, Jay Ross, Dan Salain, Yordak Salermo, Amy Sheehan, Matt Snowden, Gary Sternberg, Paul Stephens, Denise Teuber, Nicola Thomas, Lillian Vazquez, Justin Vogel, Keith Westby, Fran Wincott, Barbara Wood, Julie Yoon, Joe Deen, and our other fantastic MSLs. We would like to single out Kristine Curtiss and William "Bill" O'Connor, who were instrumental at the very beginning, helping to create the momentum that has continued for a quarter of a century. Thanks also to all the board members that David has worked with at all these companies.

In addition to scientific and technical know-how, Eyetech and Ophthotech/Iveric were strengthened by the surefooted legal maneuvers conducted by David Redlick, who provided instruction on how to navigate the complex terrain of the biotech landscape. Later, his shoes were deftly filled by Graham Robinson and Laura Knoll.

Mastery of numbers is essential in both business and drug development. David remains indebted to Marc Buyse, Robert Makuch, and Tom Fleming for teaching him statistics, a pivotal element in attaining approval.

Receiving the FDA's stamp of approval is the end point of drug development and the start of commercialization in the world's largest market. We are extremely grateful that throughout the revolution presented in this book that Wiley Chambers, until his retirement in 2024, has been the agency's watchful eye over ophthalmology and a great teacher to us all. It's vital to acknowledge the many thousands of patients who have participated in the numerous drug trials mentioned in this book. They are in every sense at the frontline of drug development, regardless of whether or not the treatments they receive are approved.

As this book makes clear, shepherding drugs through the trial process and/or successfully launching them in the marketplace is a monumental achievement. We are forever thankful to all my Eyetech, Ophthotech/Iveric, and EyeBio coworkers who have made this possible. This could not have been done without their combined efforts.

This book concludes with the acquisition of EyeBio by Merck. But that is unlikely to be the end of the story. The EyeBio team is extremely grateful to Dean Li, Eliav Barr, Joerg Koglin, Sunil Patel, and Susan Neunaber, plus the rest of the Merck team for ensuring their efforts will be taken to the next level as part of Merck, continuing the hope that even more people will have their sight saved.

Gathering ideas and experiences then putting them into words is just the beginning of book creation. Without the efforts of Amplify Publishing Group's team members Will Wolfslau, Jenna Scafuri, Jack Callahan, and editor Sarah Herse, the chapters of this book would never have been enclosed between its covers.

We are also grateful to the Gotham Ghostwriters agency's Nate Roberson, who played matchmaker bringing together three ophthalmologists with a story to tell and the son of an ophthalmologist with an attentive ear.

Writing a book—especially one like this—is far from the solitary experience so often sentimentalized in popular culture. Rooted in the companionship of David, Samir, and Tony, this book has been sustained by the support of friends and family. David is especially grateful to his amazing wife Maria and incredible sons Luca and Oliver for ensuring he remains emotionally grounded regardless of any surrounding turbulence. Their love has been fundamental to his success while supplying motivation to keep moving forward. He is also thankful for his deceased parents, Harriet and Herbert Guyer, who were always there for him and provided a source of strength. We thank Arti Patel for all her support over the years and, of course, her clever names for drugs, and Mary Adamis, who has stood by Tony as his career has shifted its locus across the North American continent. And we'd be remiss not to appreciate the steadfast Mr. Knutt and the many other family and friends, too numerous to name but vital to all our efforts.

Much appreciation goes to Ian's life partner and former *New York Times* fact-checker, Sahara Briscoe, who was the first to read every chapter. Sahara's enthusiasm and encouragement ensured progress all the way to the conclusion. Ian is eternally grateful to his father, Theo Keldoulis, the president of the Royal Australian and New Zealand College of Ophthalmology, for posthumously creating the opportunity to write this book.

—DAVID R. GUYER, MD AND IAN KELDOULIS

ABOUT THE AUTHORS

DAVID R. GUYER, MD

David is a retina specialist and a highly successful serial entrepreneur, and has been CEO of multiple public and private companies. He has seen vision research from the perspectives of academia, biotech, venture capital, and Big Pharma.

David has cofounded three biotech companies—Eyetech, Ophthotech (later known as Iveric Bio), and EyeBio—and led them as CEO. All three have been successfully acquired, with two of the companies completing huge IPOs. At Eyetech, David and his team developed and commercialized the first anti-VEGF drug for retinal diseases. He and his team negotiated an ex-US deal with Pfizer, took the company public, launched the drug Macugen, and then the company was acquired. Under David's leadership, Ophthotech entered into an ex-US partnership with Novartis that, which at the time, was one of the largest ex-US partnering transactions in biotechnology industry history. David with Samir and their team in-licensed and developed IZERVAY, which created the first class of complement inhibitors commercially available for patients with dry macular degeneration. This endeavor led to the acquisition of Iveric by Astellas for $5.9 billion in 2023.

Currently, David serves as the CEO and president of EyeBio, now a subsidiary of Merck & Co., Inc. (Rahway, New Jersey, USA). He led, with Bruce Peacock, EyeBio's acquisition by Merck in July 2024 for up to $3 billion. He is also a venture partner and former partner at SV Health

Investors, a leading venture capital firm centered on investing in healthcare innovations. David has expansive medical, drug development, and commercial experience in the field of ophthalmology, and has served on over 25 boards of both public and private companies as an independent board member, a VC board member, and CEO board member, representing all viewpoints around the board table. He has also mentored over twenty of his employees who have become CEOs.

Additionally, David has had an extensive academic career, culminating with being a professor and chairman of the Department of Ophthalmology at New York University School of Medicine. David did his undergraduate studies graduating summa cum laude and Phi Betta Kappa at Yale College. He then received his medical degree (MD) at the Johns Hopkins University and also undertook his ophthalmology residency there at the Wilmer Ophthalmological Institute before becoming a retina fellow at the Massachusetts Eye and Ear Infirmary at Harvard Medical School.

Following his medical training, David was recruited by Dr. Larry Yannuzzi (one of the most famous retina physicians of all time) to the Manhattan Eye, Ear & Throat Hospital and Vitreoretinal Macular Consultants of New York, one of the most prestigious retina practices in the world.

When he is not exploring potential new retinal therapies or starting or running new companies, David enjoys working out and has run five marathons. An avid traveler, he has been to all 50 states in the US and approximately 100 countries, where he often seeks exciting culinary experiences—especially extremely spicy foods—which he loves to share with his wife Maria and two sons, Luca and Oliver.

IAN KELDOULIS

Ian is an Australian writer who prefers shade to sunshine and crowded sidewalks to the outback. His favorite sport isn't cricket or rugby but people-watching. So, it's just as well, he's been transplanted to New York City for almost four decades.

Writing has been the one constant in his life, beginning with underground magazines while studying at Sydney University. Then he traveled to Tokyo and wrote for a local production company, Twenty-First City, and also Japanese children's TV. Work for PBS and Showtime followed when he moved to New York.

A stint in publishing led to stories in *The New York Times*, *Harper's Bazaar*, and other media outlets before he was lured into advertising, eventually running his own agency and winning ten awards for multi-million-dollar campaigns for clients such as Barclays Bank and Wine Australia. That period, along with a lot of animated dog commercials, included ghostwriting the chairman's letter for the company at the top of the World Trade Center—after hundreds of his employees were lost on 9/11. Ian continues to help businesses with complex offerings and services tell their stories to non-consumer audiences.

Recently, Ian has returned to screenwriting, and his scripts for film and TV have won numerous awards at film festivals around the world. He has also written the satirical novel, *Toyz On Demand!* about what happens to Santa Claus when the North Pole melts. Ian is now combining his years as a storyteller with his experience producing advertising to bring a slate of productions to screens large and small, with his new production company, Shade 2 Sunshine.

Ian champions causes close to his heart, serving on the board of Downey Side, an adoption agency that gives school-age foster children a chance to be in loving, permanent families. His book, *America's Youngest Hostages*, written for the organization, highlights the urgent need for reform in the foster care system. He is also on the board of the Bronx Independent Cinema Center, advocating for a vibrant cultural hub and filmmaker incubator in a borough long overlooked by the film industry.

CONTRIBUTING PARTNERS

SAMIR C. PATEL, MD

Samir is a biotech executive/consultant and retinal surgeon. Previously, Samir was the cofounder and executive chair at Kalaris, where he led the development of TH-103, a fully humanized, recombinant fusion protein from pre-clinical entity to Phase I clinical trials.

Before Kalaris, Samir was the cofounder, president, and chief executive officer of Ophthotech. Samir served as the president and vice chairman of the board of directors of Ophthotech from its IPO until January 2017. At Ophthotech, Samir in-licensed a C5 inhibitor (*Avacincaptad Pegol*). He led its development from a pre-clinical entity to the first human clinical trial for the treatment of Geographic Atrophy (GA). Subsequent trials led to the FDA approval of *Avacincaptad Pegol* for Geographic Atrophy secondary to age-related macular degeneration.

Samir was the cofounder and chief medical officer of Eyetech Pharmaceuticals, Inc., which developed Macugen from Phase 1 trials to the first approved anti-VEGF agent for the wet form of age-related macular degeneration. At Eyetech, he also served on its board of directors.

Samir has sourced, in-licensed, and led the diligence, resulting in the development of multiple new molecular entities from a preclinical compound to several multicenter, global Phase 3 clinical trials. Under his leadership, financing totaling over $310 million from private funds has been raised. As part of the senior executive fundraising team, additional private capital totaling over $200 million and four public offerings have been executed, coupled with two of the largest ex-US big pharma collaborations (with Pfizer and Novartis).

Samir has extensive experience interacting with and presenting to the US FDA on a broad range of topics. Similarly, he has had meetings and presentations with the regulatory authorities of EU member states and the CHMP advisory. Samir has also presented to the USPTO, resulting in subsequent patent issuance. Samir led and developed the clinical strategy, protocol designs, regulatory strategy, drug delivery initiatives, business development/strategy, and investor relations at Ophthotech until it evolved into a publicly traded entity.

During over a decade in academic medicine, Samir served as the director of the Retina Service and the residency program at the University of Chicago, Department of Ophthalmology and Visual Science. His area of academic interest focused on cell-based therapies for age-related macular degeneration. He was the first physician to perform a human retinal transplant.

Samir has served as a consultant to several ophthalmic biotechnology companies, healthcare venture firms, and the nonprofit entity Orbis International. He has served on the board of directors of AFER-ARVO, EyeGate Pharma, Mimetogen, and a publicly listed ophthalmic company on the Hong Kong Exchange (Zhaoke Ophthalmology). Samir has presented at numerous scientific meetings at leading ophthalmic societies, investor banking meetings, and is frequently invited to ophthalmic entrepreneur sessions.

Samir received his medical degree from the University of Massachusetts Medical School and completed his ophthalmology training at the University of Chicago. He received his training in retinal surgery at the Massachusetts Eye and Ear Infirmary, affiliated with Harvard Medical School.

TONY ADAMIS, MD

Tony is best known for his co-discovery of the pivotal role of VEGF in eye disease. Conducted at Harvard in the 1990s, this research led to his sharing the Antonio Champalimaud Award, the highest honor in vision science, and his election to the National Academy of Medicine.

At Eyetech, which he cofounded with David, and later at Roche, Tony helped lead the development of the first anti-VEGF drugs for wet age-related macular degeneration (AMD) (Macugen), diabetic macular edema (DME), diabetic retinopathy (DR), retinal vein occlusion (RVO), and myopic choroidal neovascularization (Lucentis). These drugs have significantly reduced the incidence of blindness around the world.

At Roche, where Tony served initially as vice president and global head of ophthalmology for its subsidiary Genentech, Tony helped lead the research and development of Vabysmo and Susvimo. Over almost twelve years, Tony's purview expanded to include infectious disease, immunology, metabolism, and neuroscience, culminating with him becoming senior vice president, global head of development. At EyeBio (now a wholly-owned subsidiary of Merck), which Tony also cofounded with David, he serves as chief scientific officer.

Additionally, Tony cofounded Jerini Ophthalmic which was acquired by Shire in 2008 and Aiolos Bio, acquired by GSK in 2024. Over the course of his career, Tony has helped develop 20 medicines across 30 indications, resulting in 7 Breakthrough designations and 32 FDA approvals.

Tony has also been very active in teaching ophthalmology. From 1991 to 2002 he served on the faculty of the Harvard Medical School. He also held a number of positions at the Harvard affiliated Massachusetts Eye and Ear Infirmary (MEEI), including director, residency training in Ophthalmology and co-director of its Retina Research Institute for Diabetic Retinopathy and Macular Degeneration. In 2001, he served as president of the medical staff and then became a MEEI director for 2002. Beyond teaching, Tony is the author of more than 150 scientific articles.

Tony received his MD with Honors from the University of Chicago Pritzker School of Medicine and his undergraduate degree from the University of Illinois, Urbana. He completed his ophthalmology residency training at the University of Michigan. His research training in vascular biology was at Boston Children's Hospital with Judah Folkman, MD.

After years living in Boston, New York, and the Bay Area, Tony has recently relocated with his wife Mary to Florida. He also finds time to travel, dine with friends and family, and race cars.

DAVID'S TOP 40 FAVORITE RESTAURANTS IN NO PARTICULAR ORDER

1	LA MANI IN PASTA, ROME | ITALIAN	*Cacio e Pepe and Spaghetti Carbonara*
2	DAILY CATCH, BOSTON | SEAFOOD	*Squid Ink Linguini in a Pan*
3	SCALINATELLA, NEW YORK CITY | ITALIAN	*Veal Parmigiana*
4	LA TAQUERIA, SAN FRANCISCO | MEXICAN	*Tacos*
5	JOE'S STONE CRAB, MIAMI | SEAFOOD	*Crabs*
6	LOS DOS MOLINOS, PHOENIX | MEXICAN	*Cheese Enchiladas*
7	FOGO DE CHÃO, RIO DE JANEIRO | BRAZILIAN	*Picanha with Cheese*
8	CELESTE, NEW YORK CITY| ITALIAN	*Tagliatelle con Gamberi*
9	JOE'S SHANGHAI, NEW YORK CITY | CHINESE	*Soup Dumplings*
10	FRANKLIN'S, AUSTIN | BBQ	*BBQ*
11	RITA'S CHILLI CHAAT, LONDON | INDIAN	*Chaat*
12	OSTERIA DE FORTUNATA, ROME/MIAMI | ITALIAN	*Cacio e Pepe*
13	IL MULINO, NEW YORK CITY | ITALIAN	*Veal Parmigiana*
14	FRANK PEPE PIZZERIA, NEW HAVEN | PIZZA	*Pizza*
15	ANTICA PIZZERIA DA MICHELE, NAPOLI, ITALY | PIZZA	*Pizza*
16	PEQUOD'S PIZZA, CHICAGO| PIZZA	*Pizza*
17	RINO'S PLACE, BOSTON | ITALIAN	*Lobster Ravioli*
18	JUMBO'S, SINGAPORE | CRAB	*Chili Crab*
19	FAMIGLIA MANCINI, SAN PAULO | ITALIAN	*Many Pastas*

20	**REDFARM, NEW YORK CITY | CHINESE**	*Three Chili Chicken*
21	**JAY FAI, THAILAND | THAI**	*Crab Omelette*
22	**BAR-BILL TAVERN, EAST AURORA (BUFFALO), NY | PUB**	*Chicken Wings*
23	**RED'S EATS, WISCASSET, ME | SEAFOOD**	*Lobster Roll*
24	**SPRAGUE'S, WISCASSET, ME | SEAFOOD**	*Lobster Roll*
25	**ROCKPOOL BAR & GRILL, MELBOURNE | AUSSIE SURF & TURF**	*Steak*
26	**GUS'S FRIED CHICKEN, MEMPHIS, TN | CHICKEN**	*Fried Chicken*
27	**EL CHUBASCO, PARK CITY, UT | MEXICAN**	*Cheese Enchiladas*
28	**PRETZEL BELLE, ANN ARBOR, MI | COMFORT**	*Burger*
29	**CENTRAL BBQ, MEMPHIS, TN | BBQ**	*Ribs*
30	**PIKE PLACE MARKET, SEATTLE, WA | SEAFOOD**	*Salmon Sandwich*
31	**ZORN'S , BETHPAGE, NY | HOMESTYLE POULTRY**	*Chicken*
32	**MOTHER'S, NEW ORLEANS, LA | CREOLE**	*Biscuits & Jambalaya*
33	**BOSTWICK'S CHOWDER HOUSE, EAST HAMPTON | SEAFOOD**	*Flounder*
34	**FOX BROS BAR-B-Q, ATLANTA, GA | BBQ**	*Ribs*
35	**DON JULIO, BUENOS AIRES | PARILLA**	*Steak*
36	**SEAFOOD BUFFET, DEER VALLEY, UT | SEAFOOD**	*Buffet*
37	**HARVEST ON FORT POND, MONTAUK, NY | ITALIAN**	*NY Calamari Salad*
38	**DALESSANDRO'S, PHILADELPHIA, PA | DELI**	*Cheesesteak Sandwich*
39	**LA FONDITA, EAST HAMPTON, NY | MEXICAN**	*Nachos*
40	**SZECHUAN KITCHEN (CLOSED), NEW YORK | CHINESE**	*Fond Memories*